Fighter's Fact Book 2
Street Fighting Essentials

Fighter's Fact Book 2
Street Fighting Essentials

written and edited by
Loren W. Christensen

YMAA Publication Center, Inc.
Wolfeboro, NH USA

YMAA Publication Center, Inc.
PO Box 480
Wolfeboro, NH 03894
800 669-8892 • www.ymaa.com • info@ymaa.com

Paperback ISBN: 9781594394843 (print) • ISBN: 9781594394423 (ebook)

Publisher's Cataloging in Publication

Christensen, Loren W.
 Fighter's fact book 2 : street fighting essentials / written and edited by Loren
W. Christensen.
   p. cm.
 ISBN-13: 9781594394843
 1. Martial arts--Training. I. Title.
 GV1102.7.T7C423 2007
 796.815--dc22   2016909484

The author and publisher of the material are NOT RESPONSIBLE in any manner whatsoever for any injury that may occur through reading or following the instructions in this manual.

The activities, physical or otherwise, described in this manual may be too strenuous or dangerous for some people, and the reader(s) should consult a physician before engaging in them.

Warning: While self-defense is legal, fighting is illegal. If you don't know the difference, you'll go to jail because you aren't defending yourself. You are fighting—or worse. Readers are encouraged to be aware of all appropriate local and national laws relating to self-defense, reasonable force, and the use of weaponry, and act in accordance with all applicable laws at all times. Understand that while legal definitions and interpretations are generally uniform, there are small—but very important—differences from state to state and even city to city. To stay out of jail, you need to know these differences. Neither the author nor the publisher assumes any responsibility for the use or misuse of information contained in this book.

Nothing in this document constitutes a legal opinion, nor should any of its contents be treated as such. While the author believes everything herein is accurate, any questions regarding specific self-defense situations, legal liability, and/or interpretation of federal, state, or local laws should always be addressed by an attorney at law.

When it comes to martial arts, self-defense, and related topics, no text, no matter how well written, can substitute for professional, hands-on instruction. **These materials should be used for academic study only.**

Printed in Canada.

Contents

It is not the strongest of the species that survive,
nor the most intelligent,
but the one most responsive to change.

- Charles Darwin

Introduction

Let me begin by saying thanks to the many readers who made the first *Fighter's Fact Book* a bestseller in the martial arts genre. Thanks for the nice reviews and for the kind emails over the years.

I've written quite a few books on the martial arts, about two dozen at this point. I would not have written nearly that many without the invaluable help from my martial arts pals around the world. I'm talking about the 11 writers whose work appears in this book whose combined experience adds up to over 300 years and their combined black belt ranking adds up to around 75th dan. Their street experience can only be measured in their scars and their hard-earned knowledge that they share in their books, DVDs, classes, and in this volume of *Fighter's Fact Book 2: The Street.*

As a character in one of those poorly dubbed Hong Kong chop socky flicks would say, "These guys are pretty tough guys. Their kung fu is very good." Well, for sure they are tough and some have indeed studied kung fu; mostly though, they represent a large variety of fighting disciplines that have helped them survive real world violence. Their knowledge is street tested. For some of them, it's still tested every day.

I was most pleased that my friends agreed to contribute to this book. I was pleased for my own selfish reason in that I would get to learn from them, as I have so often before. And I was pleased that their contribution, based on their experiences on the street, would make this book the highly informative one it is.

Fighter's Fact Book 2 isn't about pretend fighting at a Saturday tournament. It's not about a fun way to lose weight, a look into another culture, or any of the other things that martial arts study offers. It's about survival, plain and simple, written by martial arts veterans who know how to fight in an arena that isn't anything like the clean, open space of a training facility. These warriors can function when their pulse rate hammers at 175 beats-per-minute and when their adrenaline surges like a tsunami. They know fear and they know how to make it work for them.

I know you will enjoy this book as much as I have writing, compiling, and editing it. Read it carefully and heed its advice.

Be safe and train hard.

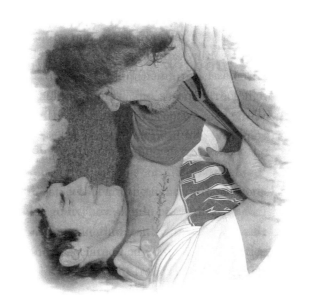

SECTION ONE
JUSTIFICATION

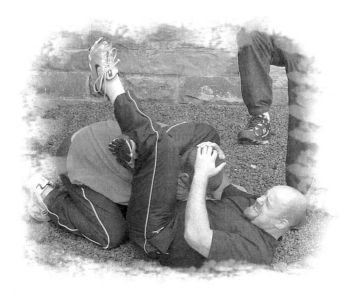

Don't Go to Jail

By Loren W. Christensen

The martial arts in general, this book specifically, contain violent techniques that run the gamut from mild pain control holds all the way to moves that can kill. Therefore, I will remind you many times throughout this book to be justified to use certain techniques and, if I did my job well, this will ingrain itself into your brain. Here is a warning in advance: *Be justified. Be justified. Be justified.*

Know and understand the law where you live. Remember, in the eyes of the law, ignorance is no excuse.

Consider this legal subsection on the use of deadly force. It happens to be Hawaii's but it's basically the same everywhere.

"The use of deadly force is justifiable under this section if the actor believes that deadly force is necessary to protect himself against death, serious bodily injury, kidnapping, rape, or forcible sodomy."

There are, of course, hundreds of variables to any situation, but taken as presented here, you're legally justified to take a life to keep yours from being seriously injured, kidnapped, raped, forcibly sodomized, or killed. Most will agree that this is reasonable. But will the police simply be okay with you saying that you believed deadly force was necessary? No. The case will be investigated and you can count on it being investigated very, very thoroughly. The facts, witness statements, and the evidence all need to support your belief. So you better be right. You better be justified.

Now, let's visit Master Tuff Guy's School of Self-defense. We're just in time for his beginner class.

A lesson in overkill

"Okay, listen up, people," 25-year-old Master Guy says. "When the attacker grabs your wrist like this, bring your arm up and over to force him to bend forward at the waist and release his grip. Now, quickly wrap your arm around his neck, and squeeze until you hear him sputter and you feel his strength fade. Now, step through hard and fast and snap his neck."

Say what? *Snap his neck!?* Because he grabbed your wrist? Seems kind of extreme, don't you think? Maybe we heard that wrong. Let's check out Master Guy's colored belt class.

"The attacker has a blade," Master Guy says, handing a rubber knife to a woman wearing a blue belt. He tells her to poke it at him. "Grab her wrist like this and bend it back to force the knife away like this. Okay, now sweep her feet out from under her. Now quickly slice the blade across her neck, once, twice, then across her stomach, once, twice, and finish by plunging it into her heart."

"Oooo" goes the class in unison. The master sure is flashy. And those deadly payback moves? Wow.

But no one in the class stops to consider this: The attacker no longer had the knife when the master butchered her. Yes, she might have another in her pocket, but that isn't mentioned in the scenario. Master Guy said, "The attacker has a blade. *A* blade. Singular. Might she have another? Sure, she might.

But you can't fillet a person for something she *might* have.

In the white belt class the new students are wowed by the nasty technique they are learning – *Awesome! We're breaking a guy's neck!* - and they look at Master Guy in awe. No one considers that Master Guy's response to the provocation is just a tad over the top. So much so that should they do that move on the street they would be doing many years in a little cell with a bunkmate named Brutus.

Are these scenarios exaggerations of what is happening in martial arts classes everyday? Not even a little bit. I've been guilty of doing it, too, but not for a long time now.

This book contains techniques for street survival that can cause pain, minor injury, serious injury, debilitating injury, and death. It's paramount that you – teacher and student – practice these techniques and any variations you devise, with responsibility and constant analysis as to the moves you're using and the imagined situations in which you're employing them. You want to consider these elements for your training partner's safety and for the legal impact they can have on you. Why do all this? Because too often we just practice defense and counters with intent to reap mayhem on our pretend attacker without considering the legal outcome had this situation been real.

Train for real in all aspects

The old axiom of *how you practice is how you will respond in a real situation* is true (for more on this see Chapter 2). If you practice an eye gouge and a windpipe choke in response to someone grabbing your wrist, then that is likely how you will respond in a real situation. Do you want to try to convince a judge and jury that that was the best way for you, a trained martial artist, to react? Well, you can try, but bring a toothbrush because you're likely going to jail. And you're going to get sued.

Karate instructor Lawrence Kane (Chapters 6 and 11) has an expression I like. "Self-defense Rule #3: Don't go to jail." A good one to keep in mind.

You might argue that you and your teacher have no intention of ever responding in such an extreme manner in a real situation where the wrist is grabbed. You say that the grab is simply a device, a stimulus, so that you can practice your counter attack – your over-kill counter attack. It's just practice. Your training partner grabs your wrist and you go postal on him, and you practice it over and over until...it's ingrained.

It's ingrained. It's fixed in your brain. Imbedded. Deep rooted.

There are thousands of schools and millions of students who practice that way.

Continuum of force

The Continuum of Force model has been used by law enforcement agencies for years, though many agencies across the country are now moving to a different one, a new and improved version called "Force Options." For the purpose of our discussion here, the Continuum of Force still works nicely.

Police

Force Options and Continuum of Force provide the police with a guideline to follow when they are compelled to respond with force in a situation. To give you a visual, think of the continuum as a ladder with several rungs. Read it from the bottom rung up.

- Lethal force (firearms)

- Impact weapons (batons)

- Defensive body tactics (hands-on tactics)

- Pepper spray (A dash of cayenne to shut down the vision and disturb the breathing)

- Passive control (physically moving a person)

- Verbal commands (voice commands)

- Officer's presence (commanding and authoritative presence)

To give you an example of how it works, I'll simplify it and make the ladder a little one with just three steps.

- On the fist rung, the officer uses his presence and voice commands to control an agitated person.

- When the subject escalates the situation, the officer moves up the continuum of force to use physical control techniques, such as wrist locks and takedowns, pepper spray, and the police baton.

- Should the subject threaten or attempt to use a weapon against the officer or someone in the officer's presence, the officer can escalate all the way up the continuum ladder to lethal force, to include extreme empty hand techniques, extreme baton techniques, or the firearm.

Now, some violent situations occur so suddenly that the officer must bypass the first rung or two on the continuum and immediately use pepper spray or the baton. Some explosive situations necessitate that the officer, within a second or two of contact with a dangerous subject, jump all the way up to lethal force.

Civilians

Civilians should also follow a continuum of force, one that is somewhat similar to that used by law enforcement. Before I get into it, allow me to say that civilians have one primary advantage that law enforcement doesn't enjoy. When there is an opportunity, civilians can move away from danger; they can run from it. However, law enforcement must move *toward* the danger. That is a huge difference that many people don't recognize.

Civilian continuum of force model Here is a simple civilian continuum I devised for discussion. Again, read from the bottom of the ladder up.

- Lethal force

- Hands on with force, including injury, to stop the threat

- Hands on with pain to control

- Hands on with little or no pain

- Strong presence and firm voice

- Voice and presence

- Avoid high-risk situations

To help see and understand the levels, let's use three scenarios in which you respond at the lowest continuum with an erect posture, a neutral expression, direct gaze, and verbiage that leaves no confusion as to it meaning. Then the scenarios are going to get increasingly more dangerous and you're going to escalate your response in kind.

Avoid high-risk situations

Follow your common sense and avoid dangerous bars, street corners, convenience stores and parks. People often get into trouble because they blunder into situations that, after the dust settles and their wounds heal, they see that their decision was not a wise one. Avoid a problem by not putting yourself into its midst.

- You know there is a bully in your school or at your job. While it's not always easy, do all that you can to avoid being around him and giving him an opportunity to intimidate you. Though you might be able to successfully fight him off, who needs the hassle?

- You see a street beggar a few yards up the sidewalk grabbing at passersby. Why put yourself at risk? Swallow your pride and cross the street. You will soon forget about it and life will be grand. But should you choose to walk by the aggressive beggar, a situation might unfold that could be costly in terms of your well-being, his well-being, court time, lawyers, and so on.

- One of your uncles is an obnoxious alcoholic and a pervert to boot. Every time there is a family gathering he grabs at you and says awful things. During the last few family events he has gotten progressively worse. Before the situation explodes, you need to talk to other family members and let them know what is going on. Maybe even tell them that you're not going to participate in family events as long as he is invited.

Voice and presence

Most high-risk situations – bullies, drunks, road ragers - can be controlled with a commanding presence, an authoritative voice tone, and well-chosen words. Accept the blame for the problem, apologize, and sprinkle lots of "sir" or "ma'am" in your talk.

Most of the time these things work. Those times they don't work is why we train so hard.

Let's proceed up the ladder using these same three characters: the bully, the aggressive beggar, and the drunken uncle.

Strong presence and firm voice

▶ A bully reaches for your arm.

• Standing straight and tall, you look at him sternly and say in a clear, strong voice, "Don't touch me."

▶ A street beggar approaches you from your side and asks for money.

• You look directly at him and say in a clear, strong voice, "Not today."

▶ Your drunken uncle at the family party says something inappropriate to you.

• You look straight at him with a stern expression, and say clearly, " "Please don't talk to me that way."

Hands on with little or no pain

▶ The bully grabs hold of your arm

- You jerk it away.

▶ The street beggar steps in close to block your path and then demands money.

- You nudge him away with your shoulder or hands.

▶ Your drunken uncle at the family party touches you in a way that makes you feel uncomfortable.

- You grab his hand and push it back toward him.

In such situations, you can use a limited amount of force to escape a grab, clear a path, and knock away an uncomfortable touch. Then you proceed on your way while making quick glances back to watch the person.

Hands on with pain to control

▶ The bully grabs your arm and resists your escape.

- You quickly maneuver his arm to where you can apply a pressure hold against his elbow.

▶ The street beggar steps into your path and slaps his hands on your chest.

- You knock his arms aside, push him into a wall and apply a control hold on his arm.

▶ Your drunken uncle grabs you inappropriately and pulls you into the bathroom.

- You knock his hands off you and push him down onto the floor.
- You sit on him and call for others to come and help.

Hands on with force, including injury, to stop the threat

▶ The bully grabs your arm and resists your escape. He reaches for your throat with his other hand

- You punch him in the chest and kick him in the groin.

▶ When you push the street beggar against a wall, he spins around before you can apply a control hold and grabs a stick from his backpack.

- Since he is blocking your escape route, you kick his knee and follow with a backfist to his ear.

▶ Your uncle bucks you off and then tries to climb on top of you.

- You grab a vase off the cabinet and whack him in the forehead with it.

Lethal force

▶ The bully absorbs your chest punch and groin kick without a flinch and pulls a knife from under his jacket. He lunges at you, nicking your arm.

- You grab his forearm, press it against his chest and then ram your fingers into his eyes.

- He screams, his eyes bleeding and squeezed shut in pain. But still he struggles to move the knife toward you.

- You slam a solid punch into his throat, which crumples him.

▶ The street beggar is only slightly phased by your knee kick and ear strike. He pulls an uncapped syringe from his tattered jacket pocket and stabs it at you.

- You grab his arm and are surprised by his incredible strength. He begins to maneuver the needle so that it pokes into your sleeve.

- You hammer fist his nose, and then sweep his leg, which drops him onto the back of his head.

▶ Hitting your perverted uncle in the head with the vase only makes him more determined. He grabs at you.

- You twist around so that your weight helps to pin his arms.

- With his head braced by the cabinet, you slam your knee into his temple to make him release you.

To reiterate, you don't have to go through all the continuum steps in progressive order. If, say, a street beggar approaches you and you respond with a firm, "Not today," and in anger he jabs a hype needle at you, it's legally permissible for you to jump to the top rung of the ladder, the lethal force rung. That is, if you can't run away.

"Avenue of escape"

Understand this legal term because not considering it can get you into trouble even when that street beggar jabs a hepatitis C-infected needle at you.

You're going to get asked in court, "Yes, the street beggar poked a needle at you, and yes you had a right to use lethal force against him with your martial arts-trained feet and hands. But answer this: Couldn't you have backed away? Could you have turned and ran? Isn't it true there was an unobstructed sidewalk behind you?"

Your heart goes *kuthunk,* and you mumble, "Uh..."

"Yet you chose...," the attorney says dramatically as he looks at each juror in the eye, "...to crush a homeless, hungry man's face with your martial arts-trained fist and trip him with some martial arts-trained move that caused the man's head to smash into the concrete."

Suddenly, your life is about to change.

Instructors: don't even joke about it

After I had been teaching the police academy for a number of years, the brass decided, and wisely so, that the instructors needed to use caution when making funny remarks about anything related to using force on someone. They were finding that some comments made in jest were coming back to haunt them.

While instructors always want their profound teachings to stick with a student, sometimes, according to anecdotal evidence, it's the wisecrack, the funny comment, the exaggerated technique that some students remember most of all.

"Now that you have your opponent's wrist locked, what do you do? You break it. Ha ha."

"Okay, you've knocked the guy down onto his back. Now, run away. But as you leave, give him a nice kick in the ear. Ha, ha"

"You've trapped his knife arm. Twist his arm so that that he stabs himself in the gut. Hey, that was so fun why not make him do it two or three times. Ha ha."

Might these little jests, underscored by humor and the mental image of the teacher's exaggerated technique, remain in the minds of some students and reappear in their actions under stress?

Yes, and that is why we were ordered not to joke around in any class that involved functioning under stress: empty-hand fighting, police baton, and firearms. Some students will only remember that you leaned on your subdued attacker's eye socket and forget that you did it for a laugh.

Important point: A private citizen has a *legal duty* to retreat. He or she must always explore evasion or escape first before getting physical.

Question, evaluate and research

I could give you dozens of examples and you could come up with dozens of: What if... Yeah, but... But can't you just... That's just not fair... So let me leave you with some advice that will not only improve your martial arts study, but just might keep you out of the slammer.

- Question what you're taught. Be polite about it but ask so that you understand how certain techniques and responses fit into the force continuum. If your teacher hasn't thought about this, your questions just might get him to do so.

- Evaluate techniques and responses. Is this technique over the top? Not enough? Does it push the legal envelope? For practice, evaluate the techniques in this book as to where they fit into the continuum.

- Research the laws where you live. Remember, ignorance of the law is no excuse. Maybe you really, really believe that it was okay to hit the guy 42 times with a brick when he pulled a knife on you. Well, just because you *thought* it was okay doesn't make it okay in the eyes of the law. Know the laws, know the continuum, and know what you can and can't do in various situations.

Perhaps you have heard the saying, "I'd rather be judged by 12 than carried by 6." While there are lots of incarcerated folks who might debate that, by questioning, evaluating and researching you give yourself one other option that is better than being carried or judged:

An informed, intelligent and highly-trained response.

Loren W. Christensen's biography appears in the "About the Author" page at the back of the book.

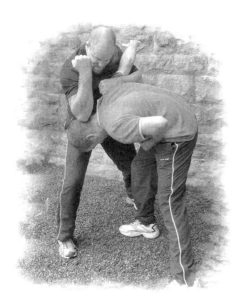 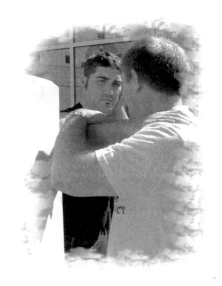

SECTION TWO
TRAINING

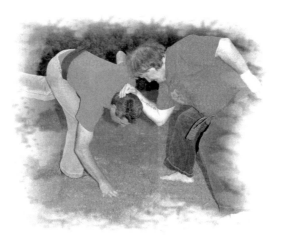

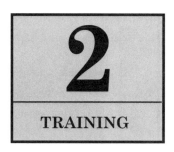

30 Questions to Ask Yourself:
You Will Fight the Way You Train

By Loren W. Christensen and Lt. Col. Dave Grossman

You will fight the way you train. I've been around the martial arts long enough to remember when no one said this now often-repeated phrase. Back in the 1960s and early 1970s, most martial artist never thought about it or, if they did, they just assumed they could alter their training to fit a real situation. Or worse, they assumed their bad training habits and methods would win the day.

While driving home after our first karate class in the summer of 1965, my buddy and I were confronted by a road rager, long before there was even the term "road rage." He pulled up along side us and threw a beer bottle at our car, missing the windshield by inches. Psyched from our introductory class, we just laughed at the bearded giant, convinced that what we had just learned would be more than enough to whip this guy into confetti. Fortunately, oh so fortunately for our dumb hides, the guy cackled madly out his window, then turned right at the light.

Over confidence is a terrible thing, and sadly, there are far too many martial artists walking around convinced that their tournament training or their aerobics kickboxing class is going to save them.

The problem isn't an isolated one in the martial arts. It's also a problem in police work and in the military. Fortunately, cops and soldiers are more aware of it now than ever and the problem continues to be addressed and fixed in their training. Also fortunately, more and more martial artists understand the concept, though, in my opinion, they are still behind cops and soldiers.

Lt. Col Dave Grossman and I wrote about this phenomenon in our book *On Combat: The Psychology and Physiology of Deadly Conflicts in War and Peace.* Here is an excerpt titled:

Whatever is drilled in during training comes out the other end in combat - no more, no less

> Whatever you would make habitual, practise it; and if you would not make a thing habitual, do not practise it, but habituate yourself to something else.
> *Epictetus (1st century A.D.)*
> *How the Semblances of Things are to be Combated*

In January 2003, Col. Grossman went to Camp Lejeune, North Carolina, to train the 2d Marine Division. He filled up the base theater twice, each time giving a four-hour block of instruction to Marines about to deploy to Iraq. "As usual," Col. Grossman says, "I taught them, and they taught me. One marine told me, 'Colonel, my old Gunny taught me that in combat you do *not* rise to the occasion, you sink to the level of your training.'"

We can teach warriors to perform a specific action required for survival without conscious thought but, if we are not careful, we can also teach them to do the wrong thing. Some trainers call these "bad muscle memory" or "training scars." They are "scar tissue" in the midbrain that is counterproductive to survival.

One example of this can be observed in the way police officers conducted range training with revolvers for almost a century. Because they wanted to avoid having to pick up all the spent brass afterwards, the officers would fire six shots, stop, dump their empty brass from their revolvers into their hands, place the brass in their pockets, reload, and then continue shooting. Everyone assumed that officers would never do that in a real gunfight. Can you imagine this in a real situation? "Kings X! Time out! Stop shooting so I can save my brass." Well, it happened. After the smoke had settled in many real gunfights, officers were shocked to discover empty brass in their pockets with no memory of how it got there. On several occasions, dead cops were found with brass in their hands, dying in the middle of an administrative procedure that had been drilled into them.

Stories like this would be hard to believe if you heard them in a bar. It is "passing strange," *indeed*, but after hearing about this repeatedly in personal interviews and seeing it in scholarly research we know that it is actually happening. In biomechanics and kinesiology this is called the Law of Specificity. In other words, you cannot get stronger legs by doing push-ups; you must train your specific leg muscles to get stronger legs.

One police officer gave another example of learning to do the wrong thing. He took it upon himself to practice disarming an attacker. At every opportunity, he would have his wife, a friend or a partner hold a pistol on him so he could practice snatching it away. He would snatch the gun, hand it back and repeat several more times. One day he and his partner responded to an unwanted man in a convenience store. He went down one isle, while his partner went down another. At the end of the first aisle, he was taken by surprise when the suspect stepped around the corner and pointed a revolver at him. In the blink of an eye, the officer snatched the gun away, shocking the gunman with his speed and finesse. But no doubt this criminal was surprised and confused even more when the officer handed the gun right back to him, just as he had practiced hundreds of times before. Fortunately for this officer, his partner came around the corner and shot the subject.

Disarm practice

When you practice gun, knife, club, and arnis stick disarms, do you hand the weapon back to you partner each time?

After reading this chapter you might want to reevaluate whether that is a good way to train.

Whatever is drilled in during training comes out the other end in combat. In one West Coast city, officers training in defensive tactics used to practice an exercise in such a manner that it could have eventually been disastrous in a real life-and-death situation. The trainee playing the arresting officer would simulate a gun by pointing his finger at the trainee playing the suspect, and give him verbal commands to turn around, place his hands on top of his head, and so on. This came to a screeching halt when officers began reporting to the training unit that they had pointed with their fingers in real arrest situations. They must have pantomimed their firearms with convincing authority because every suspect had obeyed their commands. Not wanting to push their luck, the training unit immediately ceased having officers simulate weapons with their fingers and ordered red-handled dummy guns to be used in training.

Consider a shooting exercise introduced by the FBI and taught in police agencies for years. Officers were drilled on the firing range to draw, fire two shots, and then reholster. While it was considered good training, it was subsequently discovered in real shootings that officers were firing two shots and reholstering - even when the bad guy was still standing and presenting a deadly threat! Not surprisingly, this caused not just a few officers to panic and, in at least one case, it is believed to have resulted in an officer's death.

Today, in most police agencies, officers are taught to draw, fire, scan, and assess. Ideally, the warrior should train to shoot until the deadly threat goes away, so it is best to fire at targets that fall after they have been hit with a variable number of shots. Today, there are pneumatically controlled steel targets on which photo realistic images are attached. The shooter might fire two rounds and the target falls, or the exercise can be designed so the target is supposedly wearing body armor and remains standing even after it is shot multiple times. To knock it down, the shooter must hit it in the head. Even better, in paintball or paint bullet training, the role players are instructed not to fall until they have been hit a specific number of times.

You do *not* rise to the occasion in combat; you *sink* to the level of your training. Do not expect the combat fairy to come bonk you with the combat wand and suddenly make you capable of doing things that you never rehearsed before. *It will not happen.*

There must be a continual effort to develop realistic simulations training so the warrior develops a set of skills that will transfer to reality. One two-tour Vietnam veteran put it this way.

"In Vietnam, I was always surprised to find I had done the right thing in tight situations. I sort of went into automatic and didn't think about what I was doing, or even remember it later. I'm a firm believer in training, that dull, boring 'If I have to do this one more time I'll scream' training that every GI hates. I hated it but in the end it let people like me perform in combat when common sense was telling me to run like hell."

How you train is how you will perform for real is a truism for law enforcement, soldiers and martial artists. Some martial artists adamantly object to this, saying that they would never react in a high-stress situation in such a way as the examples given above. To them I say simply, "Sorry, but your opinion is wrong. There is too much evidence to the contrary. And if you don't change your ways, you could be dead wrong."

Here are a few ways that some martial artists train that could come back to bite them on the behind:

- **Train to miss:** Punches and kicks are pulled three or four inches from their opponent.

- **Has never been hit**: Because students are taught to pull their techniques several inches short, they are not conditioned physically or psychologically to take a hit.

- **Take one, give one**: Never been trained to take a hit and respond immediately by hitting back.

- **Train to pass by or pass over the target:** High kicks are thrown so they pass over the opponent's head.

- **Ingrained ritual:** Every drill or sparring exercise is preceded with a salute (sometime elaborate), a nod, a grunt or an "ooos," and a pronounced step into a fighting stance.

- **Excessive politeness**: Accidental contact is followed by a partial salute and an apology.

- **Acknowledgement of getting hit**: A poorly controlled punch or kick hits and the recipient grabs the spot and calls time out.

- **Acknowledgement of hitting**: A punch or kick scores and the hitter raises his fist in triumph, turns his back, and walks back to his starting position.

- **Over recognition of an error:** An error in a drill receives a curse, a foot stomp, a shake of the head, or some other overt sign.

- **Stop on an error:** When a defense move misses or a takedown technique is done poorly, the action stops and everyone starts over.

- **Stop in range:** A technique is stopped for whatever reason and the attacker stays in range without doing anything.

- **Stop after one hit scores:** The attacker slams one in then stops, backs away, and basks in his glory.

- **False confidence:** Believes his weak hits that earned points in a tournament would stop a real attacker.

- **Too many Hong Kong movies:** Attacker does an excess of flippy-dippy kicks, somersaults, and tornado kicks.

- **Dropping hands within range:** Being in range with guard down and not attacking.

- **Over reliance on safety equipment**: Relying on the protective helmet to the extent that the head isn't covered well. Relying on padded hands and feet too much.

- **Telegraphing**: Excessive wind up before punching.

- **Never hitting low**: Low blows are not allowed because they are illegal in sport.

- **Targets ignored**: Grapplers struggle for a hold while the opponent's eyes, throat and groin are open and vulnerable.

- **Opponent can't punch or kick**: Grapplers defend against other grapplers who are not trained in how to throw quality kicks and punches.

- **Focus on one technique:** Over relies on his favorite technique, no matter how many times it gets blocked, misses, or fails to have an effect.

- **Hands the weapon back:** Defender disarms a knife, stick, or gun and then hands the weapon back to the attacker.

- **Doesn't consider other attackers:** Takes opponent down and then fails to look around for other attackers.

- **Doesn't get up strategically:** When moving from the ground to a standing position, he doesn't do so in a way that he could instantly defend himself.

- **Practices only in the air**: Punches and kicks are only thrown in the air and never on a bag. He has no idea what they feel like impacting something solid.

- **Always trains at the same intensity:** Never pushes for greater speed, greater power, and greater explosiveness.

- **Never trains with mental intensity**: Just goes through the motions as if they were half-hearted aerobics.

- **Doesn't "see" the opponent**: Practices in the air, on bags, and on the makiwara without visualizing an opponent.

- **Never trained all-out**: Never pushes training intensity into the anaerobic zone, that place where most fights occur.

- **Doesn't weight train:** Never uses resistance training to increase strength, explosiveness and speed.

---

*L*oren W. Christensen's biography appears in the "About the Author" page at the back of the book.

---

*L*t. Col. Dave Grossman, U.S. Army (Ret.) is an internationally recognized scholar, author, soldier, speaker, and one of the world's foremost experts in the field of human aggression and the roots of violence and violent crime. He is a West Point psychology professor, Professor of Military Science, and an Army Ranger who has combined his experiences to become the founder of a new field of scientific endeavor, which has been termed "Killology."

In this new field, Col. Grossman has made revolutionary new contributions to our understanding of killing in war, the psychological costs of war, the root causes of the current "virus" of violent crime that is raging around the world, and the process of healing the victims of violence, in war and peace.

He is the author of the Pulitzer Prize nominated book *On Killing*, which has been translated into several languages. The book is on the US Marine Corps' recommended reading list, it's required reading at the FBI academy, and at numerous other academies and colleges.

Col. Grossman's most recent book, *On Combat*, co-authored with Loren W. Christensen, is the highly acclaimed and bestselling sequel to *On Killing*.

Col. Grossman has been called upon to write the entry on "Aggression and Violence" in the Oxford Companion to American Military History, three entries in the Academic Press Encyclopedia of Violence and numerous entries in scholarly journals, to include the Harvard Journal of Law and Public Policy.

Col. Grossman is an Airborne Ranger infantry officer, and a prior-service sergeant and paratrooper, with a total of over 23 years experience in leading U.S. soldiers worldwide. He retired from the Army in February 1998 and has devoted himself full-time to teaching, writing, speaking, and research. Today, he is the director of the Killology Research Group and, in the wake of the 9/11 terrorist attacks, he is on the road almost 300 days a year, training elite military and law enforcement organizations worldwide about the reality of combat.

To read more about Lt. Col. Dave Grossman, visit his website at www.killology. com

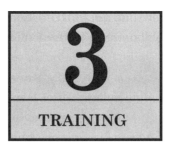

10 Ways to Make Your Sparring Street Smart

By Iain Abernethy

Almost all martial artists include sparring in their training. However, there are many different types of sparring and there is some debate as to what types are most realistic. It's even fair to say that some question if sparring has any relevance to self-protection situations. To my mind, the amount of relevance that it has to the street is determined by how that sparring is structured. With that in mind, I'd like to raise some of the key issues to consider when structuring your sparring and share 10 ways to help make yours street smart.

A word on awareness and avoidance

From the onset it's vital that you understand that fighting is what happens when self-protection has gone bad. If you are truly serious about keeping yourself safe on the streets, it's not fighting you should be focusing on, but awareness and avoidance.

The way I break down self-protection for my students is as follows: 95 percent of self-protection is awareness and avoidance skills coupled with a healthy attitude to personal safety. If you are unable to avoid a situation, you need to be able to control the dialogue and distance, strike preemptively, and use the opportunity to escape. This ability to control a situation before it becomes a fight makes up 4 percent of self-protection. The remaining 1 percent is the fighting skills you fall back on when all else fails. In my experience, it is common for martial artists to overly fixate on fighting (the last 1 percent) and hence they are not effectively addressing the issue of self-protection.

The point I'm making here is that you can be one hell of a kick-ass fighter, and yet still be incapable of keeping yourself safe. If your awareness skills are poor, you'll be taken out before you are even aware there is a threat. You simply won't get the opportunity to use your fighting skills. Consider that no matter how good a fighter you are, there will be people who are better. The way to keep yourself safe from more skilled fighters is very simple: don't fight them! Avoid the situation entirely, and if you can't, control distance through talking with your hands (keep them between the assailant and you), use dialogue and deception to facilitate a first strike, and then use the moment of confusion to flee. In this way, it can be possible to protect yourself from people you may not be able to out fight. However, if all that fails then you have no option but to fight.

As we've established, in this section we are looking at training for that last 1 percent should all your other skills fail; it is therefore not appropriate to discuss in detail awareness and pre-emption. The reason I mention them is that it is vitally important that the sparring methods we are going to examine are viewed from the correct perspective. Remember, fighting skills aren't the key to self-protection: fighting is what happens when self-protection goes bad.

Sparring and the nature of a street fight

Having established where sparring and fighting fit into the grand scheme of things, the next thing we need to cover briefly is the nature of the environment we are training for. In this book we are talking about the street and therefore the nature of the street will determine how we should spar to prepare for it. If we look at the sparring used in the various combat sports, it is immediately apparent that many differing methods of sparring exist. They vary because what is needed to win varies. What is needed to win is determined by the rules, and hence people sometimes assume that seeing as there are no rules in the street, getting rid of the rules will make sparring like a street situation. However, it's not that straight forward. Aside from the lack of rules, there are many other things that make a street situation what it is.

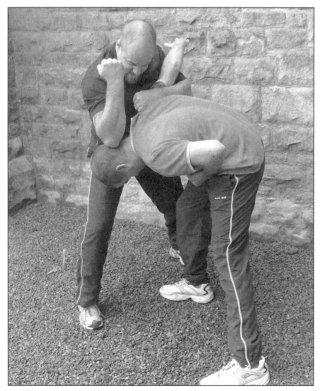

A fight is what happens when self-protection goes wrong.

The reality of street fights

A detailed discussion on the nature of street fights is beyond the scope of this look at sparring; however, here are a few key points that need to be considered:

• The vast majority take place at close-range.

• Real fights often involve multiple assailants and weapons.

• Real fights are fast, frantic and chaotic.

• Real fights do not resemble a skilled exchange between two martial artists.

• In a real situation, you need to keep things really simple.

• The fight might begin without warning (awareness being the key to ensuring it doesn't).

• Deceptive or aggressive dialogue will frequently precede any physical exchange.

• Real fights are terrifying and wholly unpleasant (assuming you're not a psychopath).

To make our sparring relevant to real situations, we need to consider all the things listed above. When they are factored in, sparring can be quite a bit different from what is seen in most dojos. This does not mean other types of sparring have no value: far from it. As a martial artist, it's very likely that you will train for a variety of reasons and have an interest in many aspects of martial training. It is therefore entirely possible that you will spar in more than one way: different types of sparring for different aspects of your training.

You may spar in one way for a straight fight with other martial artists, and another way for the street. Some argue that by sparring in more than one way you may inadvertently use the wrong method at the wrong time. I can follow this logic, but it's my view that the dojo and street environments are so radically different that it is unlikely you'll mix up the various methods so long as you keep the various types of sparring totally separate. (Almost all the leading realists that I know and train with also engage in sparring methods that aren't directly transferable to the street and yet they are easily able to keep the various methods separate.)

Having covered some of the key issues, it's now time to look at the 10 ways to make your sparring street smart.

Important point: All sparring is potentially dangerous and must always be closely supervised by a suitably qualified and experienced person. If you don't have such supervision, don't try out the methods we're going to discuss.

Be aware of the flaws of any sparring exercise

No matter how realistic sparring is, it is never real. We are always making compromises in the name of safety. If we didn't, every training session would result in the majority of students going to the hospital. We need to introduce necessary flaws into training to ensure that we can do it safely. Without these flaws, training would be just as dangerous as the street; which kind of defeats the whole point of training. It won't make our lives any safer; it will just expose us to many more life-threatening encounters.

The necessity and problem of compromise

If you do any of the following you've introduced a flaw into your sparring: train on mats, wear sparring gloves, use a gum shield [mouth guard], limit contact levels, omit techniques such as biting, eye gouges, and groin attacks, you or your partner end the fight by tapping out or submitting, and so on. Changes such as these will make training safer and more productive, but they also move it further away from a real fight. The trick to ensuring that this drift from reality is minimal is to be aware of the flaws and their effects.

By way of example, let's say you and a partner were about to engage in heavy contact sparring. To maximize safety, one precaution you may take is to wear boxing gloves. Before you start sparring, you should think about the flaws that donning them has introduced:

- Your fists are now much bigger than they would be in reality and hence your hit rate may increase.

- You can hide behind the gloves to protect yourself.

- You can't grab or effectively set up a datum and neither can your partner, meaning you use one hand to locate and control the opponent's head so the other hand can strike more accurately during the chaos of combat

- The blows have less of an effect than they would in reality.

- The nature of the gloves means that open-hand strikes cannot be delivered.

- Your grappling techniques are severely limited.

By being aware of the flaws introduced by any safety considerations, you ensure that the reality of the street stays at the forefront of your mind. Sparring is a means to an end; it is not the end in itself. Being aware of the flaws in sparring also helps keep that distinction clear.

It's not just safety that introduces flaws. You may also purposefully introduce some limitations to enhance certain skills. As an example, when sparring you may wish to isolate striking from a clinch. You limit the sparring to striking from a clinch, and therefore throws and takedowns would not be allowed. It's my observation that as soon as you limit what techniques are allowed – which can be a very useful training method – people forget about the methods that have been omitted and hence leave themselves vulnerable to them. So even if you've agreed not to permit throws when working on clinch striking, you should still ensure you don't get into bad habits by being aware of the flaw you've introduced.

Start with aggressive dialogue; not etiquette

Competitive and dojo sparring often begins with a formal show of respect. Depending on the nature of the art being practiced this may be a bow, a touching of gloves, shaking hands, and so on. Street fights don't start that way. They are frequently preceded by deceptive or aggressive dialogue. To be adequately prepared for the street, you need to have exposure to such talk so that it does not faze you.

When sparring for the street, begin the fight with one person (or more) taking on the role of the bad guy. They should close the gap with either aggressive dialogue, or deceptive dialogue that will switch to aggressive. It's important to make the dialogue and associated body language realistic. Push, shove, splay your arms, shout and swear (not in front of any kids, though). Although it's training, as the bad guy you should attempt to intimidate your partner in the same way a real assailant would.

The other person should attempt to control distance and talk the situation down. Sometimes the bad guy may decide to back away without the situation getting physical. On other occasions, either party can begin the sparring when he feels it is appropriate.

Deceptive and aggressive dialog

Deceptive dialogue occurs when the assailant closes the gap between you by asking for directions, the time, or a light for a cigarette. He appears friendly and unthreatening until it's time to become physical. Awareness, controlling distance and trusting your instincts are the key to dealing with this.

Aggressive dialogue is when the assailant screams, shouts and swears to intimidate you. The aim of this aggressive behavior is to pump himself up enough to physically attack, and to hopefully overload you with fear so that you freeze and are unable to effectively deal with the situation. If you're not used to such naked aggression, this methods will probably work and render all physical skills you have redundant.

Start without warning

Some situations will start without any warning, i.e., if your awareness wasn't what it should have been or if you are the victim of a well-executed ambush. It can therefore be good training to also have your sparring start without warning.

Sudden and unexpected sparring

Seeing as the sparring can start at any time, all participants need to wear their protective equipment throughout the entire session. The students will then engage in normal training (fitness work, drilling techniques, and hitting the pads). Whenever the leader of the training feels like it, they will shout out the command, "Fight!" At that instant all students should begin sparring with the person or people nearest to them.

The great thing about this type of training is that you are never sure what situation will develop or when. You might quickly respond to the command and attack an unsuspecting class mate, only for someone else to attack you from the rear. One second you thought you had the advantage, the next you're frantically doing your best against two opponents. After a certain amount of time, the person leading the training will shout, "Stop!" and the students return to whatever they were doing previously.

If you are training as part of a small group, another way to have sparring start without warning is to agree that anyone can attack anyone else at any point during the session (you may want to make some exceptions in the name of safety: i.e., agree that you can't be attacked when handling weights). The lack of the command to start makes the sparring all the more unexpected. It also ensures that all training done between the sparring is done with the correct attitude. If you start doing things in a half-hearted fashion, your partners may very well decide that it's a good time to attack you.

Surprise sparring is a great training method that can get you used to having to fight without warning. It is also a great way to give a training session that added edge.

Fight! Now!

It's important that the person giving out the commands does his best to ensure that the sparring is unexpected. I'm partial to shouting "Fight!" during water breaks, in the middle of drills, straight after a previous bout of sparring, while the students are performing push-ups, and immediately after I've told them the surprise sparring is over (my personal favorite). The students quickly begin to expect the unexpected and start to fight well regardless of the situation and position they find themselves in.

Keep the combat up close and personal

Most exchanges between skilled martial artists take place at a greatly exaggerated distance when compared to what happens on the street. The vast majority of real fights start close and they stay close. In the street there is rarely a gap to be closed and there is rarely any back and forth. This obviously has a significant effect on how we structure our sparring for the street.

As we've established, real situations will begin with dialogue or without warning. The distance at which words are exchanged is typically the same as punching distance. So in the case of dialogue, the distance has already been closed when the situation gets physical (people don't try to intimidate you from 15 feet away). If a situation begins without warning, then the distance has already been closed.

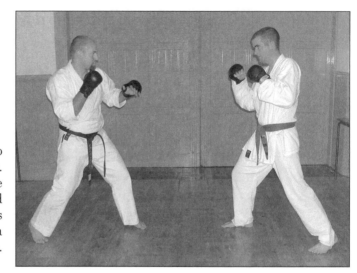

A fight is about to begin in the dojo. Notice the distance between Tim and me. Street fights take place at a much closer range.

When two martial artists fight in the dojo or competitive environment, they typically begin the fight from outside kicking distance. This means that a key part of martial arts sparring is to effectively close that gap. These skills are essentially irrelevant for the street.

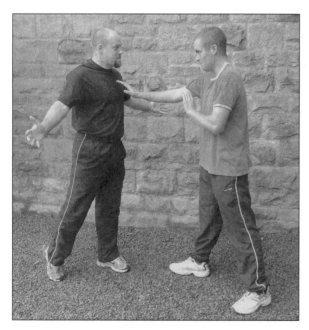

This is typically how a situation develops in the street. Here I play the bad guy as Tim takes control and lines me up for a strike. Notice how the distance has already gone before things get physical. The verbal exchange and the close proximity should be replicated in street sparring.

Another big difference between the street and a dojo exchange between two martial artists is that the there is no back and forth. In the street, people don't back off, and then move around for a bit looking for an opening before closing the gap again. All of this means that when training for the street we need to exchange techniques at close range (the exception being when we flee, which we will look at later).

Practice within arm's reach

When you start your street sparring, you should be within arms length of your partner and you should stay at that distance; with practice you'll get used to it. However, to begin with you may need to force the distance; here are two ways to do this.

- One of the best ways is to limit the floor space. The students who aren't sparring form a circle around those who are so that there simply isn't the space to exaggerate the distance.

- Another way was introduced to me by Shihan Chris Rowen. Chris simply uses a karate belt to tie the students together. It's a simple method but it works incredibly well. The students can't exaggerate the distance and hence it forces them to spar at a realistic range. The only downside with this is that the students can't practice escaping. That said, as a way to isolate close-range skills it's superb.

When you keep your sparring close there are a few things you will learn. One is that blocking becomes almost impossible. There simply isn't the time or room to react. This is a really useful learning experience as it brings home the importance of being pre-emptive and proactive in the street.

Another characteristic of close-range fighting is that it becomes very important to keep both hands active. They should be either attacking the opponent or setting him up so he can be attacked (i.e. setting datums and removing obstructions).

Keeping the sparring close is a great way to learn about what is required for the street. So to make your sparring realistic it's important to start close and stay close.

Don't bring trained responses into the mix

One of the most important things for martial artists to appreciate is that when training for the street trained responses are not a factor. As martial artists we get trained to respond in certain ways to specific stimuli, i.e. when the opponent does motion A; you are trained to respond with motion B. When two martial artists meet these trained responses are invariably exploited: martial artist 1 will move in such a way that it looks to martial artist 2 as if he is attacking with motion A. Martial artist 2 counters with motion B, just as martial artist 1 hoped he would. By responding with motion B, martial artist 2 makes himself vulnerable to motion C; which was martial artists 1's true intention. He attacked with motion A to illicit a response which would set things up for motion C.

In a street fight, you can't use trained responses in the same way; hence you need to do your best to eliminate such practices from your street sparring.

Why trained responses fail

Trained responses aren't relevant in the street for two key reasons:

• Your opponent is highly unlikely to be trained in the same martial discipline as you are and hence won't react as predicted. But what if he is a martial artist, I hear you cry.

• The street is so very different that even if your attacker is a trained martial artist he won't fight like he does in the dojo or competitive environment. Street fights are far faster, more emotional, and more chaotic than martial bouts.

Observe two world-standard martial artists fight and count the average number of techniques thrown in a 15-second period. You'll notice that most of the time is spent moving around and playing for position. The overall rate of exchange is actually pretty low. Certainly they are likely to be some blindingly fast exchanges, but they are often very short in duration. The ones that last that little bit longer are the ones when a combatant becomes injured or disorientated and the other moves in for a win.

However, a street fight is consistently frantic. It starts fast, stays fast and finishes fast. There is no time for trained responses. Indeed there is no time for responses of any sort.

In addition to being faster, a street fight is also more emotional. The intense nature of a street situation means that neither you nor your opponent will be best placed to process the information that exploiting trained responses demands. So in the unlikely event that you do meet another martial artist in a street situation, it still won't be like a dojo or competitive situation.

A good illustration of this is the fight that broke out at the Tyson/Lewis press conference in the run-up to their long awaited bout. There we had the two best heavyweight boxers at the time, but when it kicked off for real the resulting exchange was nothing like a boxing match. It was a "street fight," and was hence faster and more emotional.

Trained responses aren't a part of a street fight and hence they shouldn't be part of your street sparring. The difficulty of course is that you will be training with other martial artists so it initially takes some discipline not to engage in "game play." The instant you do start trying to illicit trained responses, you're no longer sparring realistically. In a real fight you need to keep things simple and direct. So practice keeping it simple and direct in your sparring.

Escape: Don't stay and fight!

At the very beginning of this discussion we said that a fight is what happens when self-protection goes bad. Real fights are thoroughly unpleasant affairs that can have severe medical, emotional and legal consequences. If you therefore get the opportunity to stop fighting and run you should take it without hesitation. Many a wannabe tough guy will frown on the idea of fleeing a fight, but the smart and experienced people who have "been there" will always advise flight over fight. The true warrior doesn't risk his life and liberty over his ego. He always does the smart thing.

Real life isn't a kung fu movie

I recently received an email from a martial artist who a few days previously had been approached by two men armed with knives. He quickly assessed the situation and ran away. In his email he said that he was disappointed with himself because all he could think to do was run. He asked what martial techniques he could have applied in that situation. My advice was that he shouldn't feel bad as he had dealt with the situation perfectly. His awareness was such that he had spotted the situation early enough to allow escape, and he had the presence of mind to act in what was undoubtedly the right way.

Fight two armed men and at best you're going to have some pretty big medical bills. Because he had run away, he didn't even get scratched. I'm certain that anyone who understands the street would advise nothing but running in that situation. Putting distance between yourself and a dangerous situation keeps you safe and ensures you're able to spend your time on the fun things in life. So for your sparring to be street smart, you need to practice running away.

Fleeing is more than just running

Fleeing a fight is not as straight forward as just turning tail and running. If there is a sufficient gap between you and any would be assailant, you can do just that (again, this emphasizes the importance of awareness). However, if the assailant is close enough to strike you, or the situation has degenerated into a fight, you need confusion and distance. If you don't have confusion and distance when you begin running, you will be giving the opponent your back. Bad things can occur when you do that.

If you have managed to incapacitate the opponent, even for a moment, then in that moment of confusion and disorientation you should flee. Because the opponent won't be able to immediately react, you have the chance to generate sufficient distance to allow a successful escape. When a gap appears in the street, your self-protection training should have conditioned you to make it bigger. Much bigger! You should not be thinking of closing the gap and continuing the fight.

A great way to practice fleeing in training is to make part of your dojo a "safe zone." Your aim is to reach this safe zone while your partner (or partners) prevents you from doing so. The full range of martial techniques are allowed, but if a gap is created (they rarely appear on their own) the aim is to extend it and make it to the safe zone.

Another good way to practice escaping is to have two people at either end of the dojo, while the person practicing fleeing is in the middle. The middle person will run towards the first person and they start sparring (using both grappling and striking). As soon as the fighting begins, the person who started in the middle must break contact and create a gap. He then runs to the other end and repeats the process. This drill is a great way to develop the skills needed to create a gap, and engrain the habit of running when you have the opportunity. It's also one fantastic workout.

Running away is the smart and practical thing to do whenever possible. Hence, you need to ensure fleeing is included in your sparring.

Don't limit the techniques or ranges

In a real situation, anything goes and hence you need to ensure your street sparring isn't limited. If your background is in a striking system, ensure that you bring grappling into your sparring. Likewise, if your background is in grappling, ensure that you bring striking into your sparring. The more wide-ranging you make your sparring the more realistic it will be.

Allow banned techniques

You also need to ensure that you include the techniques not allowed by the rules. In combat sports, there are two groups of techniques that will be banned. First, there are those banned in the name of the purity of the sport, i.e. boxing is about punching so anything that can stifle the exchange of punches is prohibited. All combat sports have similar restrictions in order to maintain the purity of the sport and give the spectators what they want to see. Secondly, there are the techniques that are banned in the name of safety, such as low blows. All of these banned techniques are allowed in a street situation.

Modifying dangerous techniques

A real fight has no rules, and hence you need to ensure you ignore the rule book of your art when you structure your street sparring. It's pretty easy to ignore the purity-based restrictions, but great care needs to be taken when ignoring the safety-based ones. In some instances you can substitute dangerous techniques for less dangerous alternatives. For example, if your partner secures a grip on the knot in your belt, it's a safe assumption he could also have attacked your groin in the same fashion. Likewise, putting the thumb on your partner's forehead above the eyebrows can be used as a substitute for eye gouges.

Substitutions like these ensure that you develop the skills to use and defend against such attacks. The flaw in this training is that if you're not mindful of the intent of the substitution, you may find yourself using the substitution in the street at a time when you should be using the real technique. As I said at the very start, always be aware of the flaws of any drill. Because the alternative is to omit the techniques completely, I feel substitution is the best way forwards.

In addition to substitution, you can also reduce the intensity of certain techniques to ensure safety. For example, if you nip your partner with your teeth, he can be sure he would be missing flesh if the fight was for real. It is important that your sparring is closely supervised by a suitably experienced and qualified person when bringing potentially dangerous techniques such as biting and gouging into your sparring. The person supervising the sparring will be able to advise you on substitution, omission and intensity.

By not limiting the techniques or ranges of your sparring, you ensure that "blind spots" don't develop and that your sparring has relevance to a real fight.

Emphasize simplicity & high-percentage skills

It is vitally important in the street to keep things very simple. The simpler a technique is, the more likely it is to succeed. The more complex a technique is, the more likely it is to fail.

However, it doesn't always work that way in a dojo or competitive bout between two martial artists. In that environment, using complex and sophisticated methods can catch your opponent off guard. The simple methods will be more easily recognized and countered so it can be advantageous to use methods that are "off radar." In almost all combat sports, much of what was winning fights a few years ago is now obsolete because it is easily recognized and hence easily countered. Competitors need to enhance, disguise, and evolve their techniques if they are to keep winning. Complex and indirect can work fine in the dojo or in sport. The complex and indirect won't fare well in the street, however.

Advanced isn't always better

When sparring for the street, be sure to stick to the basics. Many martial artists inadvertently associate the term "advanced" with "better." That is not how it works in the street. There is the basic stuff that works; and the advanced stuff that doesn't work. There are no such things as "advanced self-protection" or "advanced street fighting." When sparring for the street, keep everything simple and avoid any temptation to get clever.

Use fight-stopping techniques

It is also important to emphasize techniques that will have the greatest effect. A head shot will have a greater effect than a strike to the body. A strangle will finish the fight, but a joint lock might not (you can't fight when you are unconscious, but you can fight with a broken joint). Methods such as body shots and joint locks still have a role to play, but priority should always be given to the techniques that will end the fight the quickest.

For street sparring, stick to techniques that are simple, have the best chance of working, and are likely to have the greatest effect.

Vary the numbers (real fights aren't always one on one)

This is a big one. Dojo and competitive sparring is almost always one on one. Street situations aren't like that. They can be one on one but they can also be loads of other things. It's therefore very beneficial to mix up the numbers when sparring for the street.

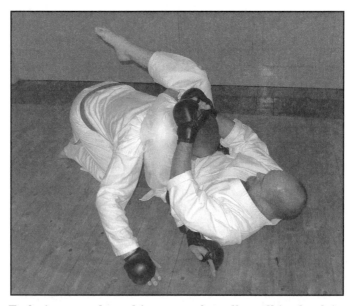

Techniques such as this can work really well in the dojo or competitive arena where the fight is guaranteed to remain one on one.

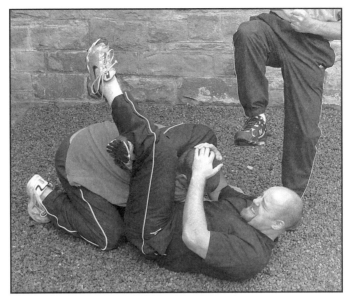

Real situations frequently involve more than one person, Sparring with multiple opponents will teach you which methods are most suitable for the street. If you do go to the ground in a street situation, don't try to finish the fight from there. Do your utmost to quickly regain your feet.

Fighting vs. protecting yourself

Successfully fighting off two or more assailants isn't anywhere near as easy as depicted in the martial arts movies. With enough commitment and ferocity, it is possible to take on more than one person successfully, but it is never advisable to do so.

The subject of multiple opponents is frequently overlooked in the martial arts world with most training focusing on the one-on-one scenario. Practicing against multiple opponents will help prepare you should the worst happen. Such training also brings home some really important lessons about how you should face street situations. Some martial artists attempt to justify the lack of training against multiple opponents by stating that successfully outfighting multiple opponents is impossible. It is true that outfighting committed multiple opponents is extremely difficult (not impossible); however, it should also be understood that you don't need to outfight them in order to protect yourself.

A few years ago, I was teaching street-based sparring drills to a mixed ability group. As part of this session we were practicing two-on-one sparring. At one end of the room was a young, relatively inexperienced martial artist who was visibly nervous at the prospect of having to simultaneously face two opponents. At the other end was a group of extremely experienced martial artists. The members of this group had multiple black belts and were all skilled fighters. This group was actually excited at the prospect of getting to test their skills against two opponents.

When I signaled for the fights to begin, the experienced martial artists went off with all guns blazing ... but invariably were quickly taken off their feet and beaten up by their colleagues. By contrast, the inexperienced martial artist did not want to test his skills. He wanted out of there! He ran all around the dojo and hardly had a punch land on him.

The moral of the story is that when faced with more than one person, don't stay and fight them but instead run away the instant you can. As I said earlier, you don't need to outfight multiple opponents to protect yourself from them. Sparring with multiple opponents really brings this lesson home and lets you practice your escape skills.

Spar two to understand how to spar one

Sparring with multiple opponents also teaches you a lot about how you should face a single opponent in the street. What begins as a one-on-one situation in the street or bar can quickly escalate. Criminals frequently work in gangs; just because you can't see them doesn't guarantee they are not there.

As an example of how the possibility of multiple opponents changes things, let's briefly discuss ground fighting. In the dojo taking the opponent to the floor and trying to finish the fight on the ground can work great. However, if you use the same methodology in the street, a second person could get involved and you would get stamped flat. Fights can go to the ground so it's something you need to include in your training and sparring, but it's never the smart choice in the street.

A friend of mine was once mugged at an ATM by what he initially thought was just one person. He's a big guy and told the mugger to leave him alone (well, that's not what he said, but Loren Christensen's writer's guide said no swearing). At that point the mugger pointed across the road where his previously unseen colleague opened his jacket to reveal a huge knife. My friend wisely decided to hand over his cash. He could also have hit and run, but I feel he undeniably made the smart choice. However, what would have happened if he'd decided to fight? Or worse yet take the fight to the ground? I think we can safely say that the initial one on one exchange would not have stayed that way for long and my friend would have been stabbed.

In your street sparring be sure to play with the numbers: one-on-two, one-on-three, two-on-three etc. You'll learn a lot about how to approach real situations.

Spar when exhausted

Real situations are very stressful. Your heart rate will go though the roof, you may feel nauseous, your muscle control will be greatly reduced, you will want to be anywhere else on Earth, and you may feel frozen to the spot. Being mentally and physically able to deal with these sensations is a key part of preparing for the street.

A good way to recreate these sensations is to fight a fresh opponent when you are exhausted. I don't mean a little bit tired, I mean exhausted! Your heart rate will be high, you may feel nauseous, your muscle control will be greatly reduced, you will want to be somewhere else and you won't feel like fighting. Not wholly unlike a street situation.

There are a great many ways to exhaust yourself. You can do some intense exercise before sparring, do a lot of pad work, or just spar back to back with a number of fresh opponents. However you go about it, sparring when exhausted should be part of your street sparring. You may not want to go to extremes every session, but you should do it frequently enough that you get used to functioning under stress. If you don't get used to it, all the skills you posses will be rendered redundant by the intensity of the situation.

There are lots of different ways to spar and all have value. Most martial artists train for a wide range of reasons aside from self-protection. However, when training for the street, it is important that your training methods accurately reflect the nature of street situations. I hope the 10 tips we have discussed will help you structure your sparring in a way that is as realistic as possible.

Iain **Abernethy** is one of the UK's leading exponents of applied karate. His numerous martial arts DVDs and books have sold worldwide and have been translated into several languages. Iain holds 5th dan black belts with Karate England, the official governing body, and with the British Combat Association, one of the world's leading groups for self-protection, close-quarter combat, and practical martial arts. Iain is one of the few within the British Combat Association to hold the position of Coach; their highest instructor qualification.

Iain regularly writes for all the UK's leading martial arts magazines and he is a member of the Combat Hall of Fame. He is in great demand on the seminar circuit where he teaches his practical approach to the martial arts both in the UK and overseas.

Iain's website is an extremely popular resource for the practically minded martial artist. In addition to numerous articles, a popular message board and free e-book downloads, the website also has a free monthly newsletter which currently has over four thousand subscribers. Check it out at www.iainabernethy.com.

Thanks to Tim Kendal for posing as the attacker and to Fred Moore for his outstanding photography.

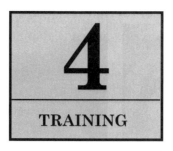

TRAINING

10 Concepts to Adapt Your Training to the Street

By Rory A. Miller

It's not enough to say that "the street" is different from the dojo. The street is different from the street. Real conflict happens in places, times, and with people. It happens for a reason, though the victim may never know what that is. The aggressor has motives, history and a plan. The professional violent criminal is one type of aggressor or threat. He has a system that he has developed through trial and error to safely and effectively neutralize you to get what he wants. There are many types of threats, and each type and each situation might require different skills.

You might be required to stop an elderly schizophrenic patient from trying to leave the nursing home. Since this is not the same kind of threat that a professional predator presents, it requires different techniques, tactics, and mindset.

A drunken relative who insists on driving is a different threat than a mob trying to flip and burn your car. A date-rape is a different threat than a bar fight. Next to surprise, the chaos and variability of real life is the hardest factor to train for.

When you bow into your dojo or shake hands at the start of a match, you know where you are, what the goals are, what to expect, and what it takes to win. In this sense, martial arts training is unitary. Whether you study arnis, judo or mixed martial arts (MMA), you're studying to a single context.

It can get really messed up when what you're training for (say, winning the next submission grappling tournament) doesn't match what you *think* you're training for ("I'm learnin' to fight.") Believing that you already have the answer to a problem not only limits your adaptability in seeking other answers but can prevent you from clearly seeing what the problem really is.

There will be tons of good advice and hard-won lessons in this book about the street: things to do, things to notice, and mistakes to avoid. The goal of this chapter is to look at your training and see it a little differently.

Concept 1: the tactical matrix and complexity

There are four ways a fight can happen:

1) You're surprised: you're the victim of an ambush.

2) You were suspicious: you knew something was happening but you weren't sure what.

3) It was mutual combat: you knew there was going to be a fight and you were ready.

4) You attack with complete surprise

There are three levels of force available that may be appropriate:

1)   It's not okay for you to cause damage.

2)   It's okay for you to damage but not to kill.

3)   It's justified for you to kill.

A matrix is a way of looking at how several elements can combine to change a situation. If you look objectively at your training, you can plug everything into the matrix and see where it's appropriate and where it's useless. Each technique, each tactic and each strategy fits somewhere in this simple box.

	SURPRISED	ALERTED	MUTUAL	ATTACKING
NO INJURY				
INJURY				
LETHAL				

Placing just these two variables, "level of surprise" in the horizontal column and "acceptable force" in the vertical column, creates a 3x4 matrix with 12 possible combinations.

	SURPRISED	ALERTED	MUTUAL	ATTACKING
NO INJURY				
INJURY				
LETHAL			Fencing	

I fenced in college. As it was taught, fencing (without the safety equipment) would only be appropriate in the Mutual/Lethal box. Can you modify this? Sure, I could always stab someone from the shadows with my epee, expanding to the lethal/attacking box, but that wasn't how it was taught.

Strategy can also be placed on the matrix. For example, the essence of karate is to close the distance and do damage. We can argue about the lethality of the fist, but in general, striking is about damage. We can also argue whether or not strategy can be useful under surprise, but for sure if it's not practiced under conditions of surprise, it won't be.

Sosuishitsu-ryu jujutsu was designed for a last ditch effort to survive an assassination attempt, or when a combatant's weapon was broken on a battlefield. It's a brutal fighting system, one designed specifically around dealing with situations of surprise and disadvantage. But it generally sucks for mutual combat or attacking; that's what swords and spears were for.

The defensive tactics (DT) I was taught at the police academy were based on taking a threat down and handcuffing him without injury. We were also trained in firearms, the Big Equalizer.

Comparative strategy matrix:

	SURPRISED	ALERTED	MUTUAL	ATTACKING
NO INJURY			DT	DT
INJURY	Sosuishitsu	Karate	Karate	Karate
LETHAL	Sosuishitsu	Sosuishitsu Handgun	Handgun	Handgun

Notice that there are few or no strategies for surviving an ambush without causing injury. That is a simple fact that is hard for some people to stomach. Surviving an ambush is difficult. When you're hampered with restrictions on how you're allowed to survive it becomes even harder.

When you consider your training, look to see where it fits in the matrix. Can you execute a trap when you're surprised? Can you justify using your reverse punch to get a senile grandparent to quit swinging his cane at the nurse?

Dojo training is much, much simpler than real violence. The matrix is a way to show that. In a simple list of 12 possible contexts for violence, it's rare to find a style, strategy or technique that is appropriate for more than three. This is just a taste, because this matrix is far too simple. You could add an entire dimension with any variable you choose to consider.

Consider weapons. There are four ways weapons can come into a fight:

1.   The defender has a weapon.

2.   The attacker has a weapon.

3.   Neither has a weapon.

4.   Both have weapons.

These four possibilities quadruple the size of the matrix. It would now contain 48 boxes in three dimensions.

Each uncontrolled element of the context of the fight expands the skills and knowledge needed and removes it farther from the unity of training.

Concept 2: Know what is going on and make a decision

Self-defense situations develop quickly. One key skill is the ability to decide what to do in an instant - then do it. If you're ambushed, you will probably take damage before you're even aware that you're in a fight. Planning takes time and on the receiving end of an ambush, time is damage. All possible solutions involve moving: either running or fighting. You will make that decision in a fraction of a second with only partial information. Each second you spend gathering information to make a better decision is a second of injury to you. Damage makes it harder to implement your plan.

If you're going to run, run. If you're going to fight, fight. If you're going to talk, talk. Keep your decision simple. If you decide to fight, then fight. Don't think: *"I must pass-parry the probable overhand right, side step to his dead zone and apply pressure to his chin and grab his shoulder, then pirouette..."* Detailed plans fall apart under chaos. Simple plans don't. Not as much.

Make a decision, make it fast, and act.

Concept 3: Discretionary time

How a person uses discretionary time is the defining difference between a professional and an amateur. To put it as simply as possible: if you have time to think, think. If you don't have time to think, move.

The people who get stomped are the ones who felt something hit them from behind, and then they froze for a second to either figure out what was going on or to make a plan. Should this happen to you, the fact that you're under attack is all the 'what' you need to know. Each second of planning or thinking is one more second of damage.

Conversely, if something is about to go bad but hasn't yet you have time to think and plan, to evaluate options, available weapons and allies, and to look for escape routes. The more time you have and the better you use it, the more power you have, not only in any eventual fight, but in deciding if one is even going to happen.

Ways to get more time

The earlier your warning systems go off, the more time you have to make a good decision. Here are some simple ways to fine-tune your early-warning systems and buy some time.

- Trust your intuition. If the hair stands up on the back of your neck, start looking for weapons, escape routes and threats *before* you try to figure out what is causing the reaction. If you don't trust someone, think about how to get away or what you will do if they lunge at you before you try to rationalize your distrust.

- Make a habit of studying your surroundings. Always look for good escape routes, obstacles, and available weapons. Practice looking for subtle reflective surfaces and shadows until it becomes second nature.

- Learn all you can about how violence really happens and how criminals really work. Choose your sources wisely - there is a lot of bad information available.

In a mutual fight, you have great discretion to set the terms of the conflict. There is a predictable build up with easily recognizable steps. I call it the "Monkey Dance," the human dominance display. The Dance can usually be averted by showing submissive body language (eyes down and an apology), or it can be circumvented by jumping steps, such as taking the threat down as he approaches, instead of waiting for the chest push.

More important is to realize that if you're aware that something is building to a fight, you don't have to agree to take it there.

Threat: "I'm gonna kick your ass."

Me: "No."

Threat: "What do you mean, 'No?' ?"

Me: "Just no."

Threat: (hyperventilates a little) "What are you gonna do about it?"

Me: (sigh or yawn [I've done both]) "Look, it's late and I'm tired. You already sound upset. Fighting would wake me up a little but I don't see what you'd get out of it. What's your goal here?"

Threat: "My goal? You're a weird cat, Miller."

Me: "I hear that a lot."

The Monkey Dance

Animals do not fight within their own species the same way they attack prey or defend themselves from predators. Big horn sheep slam the hardest parts of their heads together in dominance games, but fight off coyotes mostly by kicking. Coyotes, on the other hand, snarl, posture and wrestle to get a grip on an exposed throat of another coyote, but they prefer to run a deer or sheep to exhaustion, slashing at its hamstrings and belly with their teeth.

Though it looks like a fight, the dominance game played within a species is nothing like predatory violence. The same is true for humans. Like any other animal, humans have a ritual combat they play with other humans to establish dominance.

The steps may differ by culture but in general the Monkey Dance follows:

1) Eye contact with a hard, challenging stare.

2) Verbal challenge: "What you lookin' at?!"

3) The person closes the distance with a strut, his chest stuck out.
   Sometimes they actually bounce up and down like a rooster.

4) A push or finger poke, usually to the chest. A finger poke on the nose will almost always result in an immediate swing.

5) A hard overhand swinging punch.

It's rare for someone to be seriously injured in the Monkey Dance. Injuries that do occur happen when one or both of the participants fall and hit their heads.

The Monkey Dance may start with a clear aggressor or a bully, but as soon as the other person responds, both are involved in the dance. When challenged in this manner, most people will respond following the same steps as the aggressor unless they are aware of it and disciplined not to do so.

Concept 4: Fight to the goal

In a martial arts tournament, you know exactly what constitutes a win: a throw for *ippon* (point), a knockout, or a tap out. What determines a win is decided before the battle and is predictable enough that you can train toward it.

It's rarely that predictable in real life. The tactical matrix illustrates that fighting at different levels of force – restraint, damage, lethal - changes everything. A situation that requires you to restrain without hurting is completely different in presentation, options and goals than one that requires you to break a limb or to kill. It's incumbent on you to recognize as early as possible which situation you're in, and fight to that goal.

It would be easy if those were the only three possible goals. They aren't. What you need to prevail (your goal) in each given situation may be wildly different.

You may need to fight your way *past* someone or several people to escape, which is different than standing and fighting. You may need to get your daughter or pregnant wife to safety. You may need to get the attention of near-by help. While curled into a ball being kicked from all sides, you need to stay calm and conscious long enough to poke 9-1-1 on your cell phone. During the ensuing battle, you might need to get one hand free to access a weapon. Whatever the goal in that instant, you must fight toward it and it must be the right one.

Example of an inappropriate goal

Several years ago, I debriefed a corrections officer after a use-of-force incident in which he had been attacked by a single inmate in a large open jail room with 64 other inmates watching. He was several minutes into the fight before he realized the inmate was trying to kill him: biting, striking and gouging the officer's eyes. But the officer was only trying to go for a pin! He had been a competitive wrestler and his training had taken over. He had fought to an inappropriate goal and it could have cost him his sight or his life.

Concept 5: Use your environment

Most martial arts are practiced in an incredibly sterile environment: the floor is even and often padded, and sharp edges and corners have been removed. There's no furniture to trip over, much less puke to slip in, or needles to roll over. The practitioners are stripped down to similar uniforms with sensible (or no) footwear.

The real world is full of curbs, doorknobs, furniture, and sharp-cornered concrete buildings.

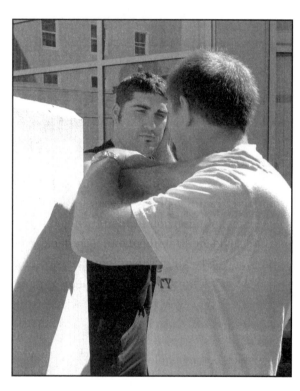

It's possible to drag someone off balance by their hoody, or blind them by pulling it over their eyes. You can immobilize a person lying on the ground by standing on their baggy pants. There are slopes and slippery places, and places where there isn't enough room to turn around. There's bad lighting, loud noises, shadows, and reflections everywhere. All the while traffic whizzes by.

The difference between a hazard and an opportunity is determined by who recognizes and exploits it first. A curb is a hazard if the threat makes you trip over it; it's an opportunity if you push him over it. The list of potential opportunities is endless.

Reading about this isn't enough. Thinking and visualizing isn't enough. You need to practice your art in a variety of surroundings and deliberately use the environment in conjunction with your art. It takes a good amount of skill and a teacher who understands safety, but you need to *practice* recognizing when walls, corners, tables, electrical cords, random liquids, the threat's clothes, and traffic can be used to your advantage. This can be dangerous. Even training in armor won't help much should you throw someone into the corner of a table.

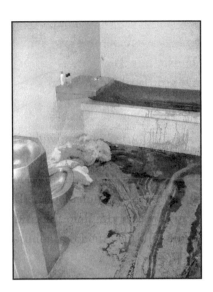

There is a big difference between this blood-smeared jail cell where officers had to fight a combative prisoner and that of the clean, sterile, and wide-open training area of a martial arts school.

Don't let the sterility of the class environment blind you to available options. Use the mirrors and the weapons on the wall. Run for the door and yell for help in self-defense class.

Want to know one of the differences between rolling with your pals at the dojo and rolling with a tweaker (someone under the influence of methamphetamines) in an isolation cell? Hygiene. Your dojo pals don't stink. Not like a tweaker.

Concept 6: Violence is a form of communication. So *communicate*

Cops often come into the job believing the Old West version of the gunfight and the quick draw. They pay lip service to the adage that "action beats reaction," but they don't really grasp it.

During "uncontrolled environment" training, officers participate with a full complement of safe weapons, including Simunitions (Sims are sub-caliber weapons, real guns that fire a marking pellet. The suckers sting, too. Ask to see the scars some time).

To demonstrate the action/reaction gap, I let two officers draw their weapons and point them at my chest with their fingers on the trigger. I have a Simunitions weapon in my hand dangling at my side. The officers are instructed to order me to drop the weapon, and should I make a threatening gesture, they are to fire. I consistently get off three shots before either officer can squeeze the trigger. If I sidestep with the action, they miss.

Then I have one of the students play the threat and I play the officer. The kid expects me to draw down and give commands. Instead, I *scream*, "Drop the weapon, do it now!" while leaping at him, grabbing his shoulder with my off hand, and spinning him to the ground. Not one trainee has fired a shot (except for the time I slipped like an idiot and fell). This demonstrates how action beats reaction, and the scream is key.

When you fight, scream and make it a sharp, loud, and simple command: "Stop!" "Get down!" "Drop it! Try to hurt his ears and shake the windows across the street.

Concept 7: This is not a game

There are no OSHA (Occupational Safety and Health Administration, a government organization that ensures safe and healthy working conditions) regulations for an assault. When a boxer isn't wearing competition gloves and he hits a skull, he breaks his hand. If you hit a threat in the mouth out in the street, you risk getting blood poisoning when broken teeth puncture your skin and his blood and saliva get into your body. Even if it's only the other guy who does the bleeding, you sometimes wait for weeks for blood tests to know if you were exposed to hepatitis or HIV.

Those are the *winning* options. The loser may be paralyzed, blinded or permanently brain damaged. It's easy for some people to say that they would risk their life for X, but the question is would they risk becoming a paraplegic and having to wake up to the same nightmare every day? Would they risk spending years in prison? Losing their house as part of a civil suit?

These are just some of the things at risk. It's not as clean as is the romantic fantasy about dying heroically for a good cause. The stakes are too high for it to be a game.

Get them talking

This is a trick I picked up yanking combative bad guys out of cells, a situation in which the prisoner is ready to fight and you have to go through a door to put him down without hurting him. He knows from what direction you will be coming and that you will be moving directly through his prime striking range.

I use a fast lead hand and lead-leg drop-step to grab just above his lead elbow. Then I spin him. The trick is to make the move while he is talking so that he freezes.

This has been so reliable that now when I know I have to take someone out of a cell and I have a few seconds of discretionary time, I try to get the person talking. Then I move.

In training, there's an emphasis on good technique and doing things right. "Start over," sensei says. But there aren't any do-overs outside the dojo. Sometimes you screw up, sometimes it's sloppy. Tough. You work from where you find yourself because that's all you have. You need to practice recovering from a position of disadvantage; accept mistakes as something that happens and work from the flawed position.

Fighting is too damn sloppy to be a game.

There are also habits in every style that are based on safety or entertainment that have become the "right" way to do the technique. Officers and soldiers put prisoners face down for control, wrestlers and judoka put them face up because it makes for a more entertaining and challenging match. The follow-through for a judo hip throw is taught as a control maneuver to get an easy pin or arm-lock, but it was a safety modification from the older follow-throughs that put the thrown person's falling weight directly on the point of his shoulder or bent neck. The pronated fist of karate was a Japanese innovation to decrease the training injuries common to the original Okinawan art. Over time these safety and entertainment changes have become the "right way" and "good technique." Study your training for things that have been added to make it safer or "more fun."

Breaking the turtle

The turtle is a defensive position common to most grappling styles. The opponent is on hands and knees, facing the floor, back rounded to use the abdominal muscles to best advantage in resisting being lifted or straightened. In styles where uniforms are worn, the turtler's hands are often inside the collar so he can protect himself from strangles. This position isn't a fight-winner, but it's a solid defensive position where an opponent can rest and think.

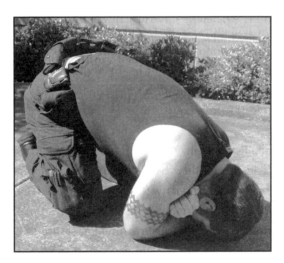

I've spent hours learning different ways to break the turtle. I'm partial to a trailing arm flip over strangle, but truth is it's a useless move. Imagine you're in a bar brawl and someone turtles up. So what? A guy curled up and face down is not a threat. If he reaches for a weapon he becomes a threat, but you do *not* engage by grappling him. You leave. Or you use a weapon of your own. Or you apply your boots to him.

The exceptions are law enforcement and corrections officers who have to handcuff a threat from the turtle position. But even then there is usually time to bring more people or tools into play.

Concept 8: Intent, means and opportunity

For a person to be seen as a valid and immediate threat, he must exhibit three elements: intent, means, and opportunity.

- Intent means that he wants to hurt you.

- Means is his ability to hurt you: fists, knife, or gun.

- Opportunity allows him to reach you with the means.

To claim self-defense, the threat must present all three of these elements and you must be able to explain clearly how you knew all were present.

If you can take one of these away, he ceases to be a threat. If you can physically beat him up you deny him his means. If you can get away, he is denied his opportunity. If you can change the threat's mind, you have altered his intent. Altering intent is a broad and potent skill. You can do it by projecting calm, bluffing, using humor, emitting an ear splitting scream, and a number of other ways.

The art of fighting without fighting

Besides attacking a threat physically, you can attack him mentally. You can attack the relationship and you can attack the context.

Attack mentally   This is a direct attempt to influence his mind. For example, loud and unexpected noises can freeze the mind for a second. So can non-sequiturs, odd phrases that make the threat reevaluate the situation.

On one occasion we had a large, violently psychotic inmate screaming threats. When he took a breath, I said softly, "I know. But you tried really hard and you did well for a long time. No one can ever take that away from you. I'm proud of you." He let me cuff him.

Attack the relationship   To do this you must understand what dynamic you're in. You and the bad guy are both playing a role, so if you change the one he has assigned to you, you change the relationship.

Threat: "What you starin' at?"

Me: "Sorry, man. Worked a double yesterday and I zoned for a minute. How you doin'?"

Attack the context   This requires a global awareness: you must know what is going on and what the threat *thinks* is going on. If he is attempting to put on a show for his friends, try to remove the friends. If a predator believes you're alone and vulnerable, start talking to someone out of the threat's line of vision or make a cell phone call. My personal favorite is this: when the threat sees me as a potential victim and I have a three-way conversation with Jesus and Elvis while rhythmically twitching, the threat tends to change his mind.

Concept 9: You won't have your normal mind or body

Remember the first time you asked someone out on a date? Your mouth was dry, your palms were sweaty, your knees felt weak, and you were unbelievably clumsy. After hours or days of working yourself up to it you were still barely able to stammer out the words. Compare that high anxiety moment to having a casual chat with your friends.

Your fighting skills in real life will degrade about as much as your verbal skills did when asking that person out. This subject can get complex.

As the stress hormones hit your system, your perception can alter:

- You might not be able to hear anything

- Your eyesight might become incredibly acute but without peripheral vision, or just a blur.

- You might not be able to feel anything with your fingers.

Your mind will alter:

- You might lock onto an idea and, though it's not working, you're unable to do anything else.

- Everything might appear to be in slow motion, but still you can't move.

- You might feel calm and peaceful as horrible things happen to your body, or to a friend's, and you don't feel like doing anything about it.

- You might meekly obey when you know you shouldn't. Many victims of horrible crimes comply simply when ordered to or when they are only threatened with violence. I had a 400-pound veteran jailhouse fighter meekly get on the ground when ordered just because of volume, intensity, and surprise of the command. I never had to touch him.

Important point: a training environment that emphasizes instant obedience to any authority figure or shouted command may make the students *more* vulnerable to this kind of assault.

Your body will alter:

- Your finger dexterity might be gone (loss of fine-motor skills).

- You might not be able to move your arms and legs at the same time (loss of complex motor skills)

- Your limbs might feel heavy or numb.

After putting a 240-pound jail guard through a scenario that was an emotional wringer, he leaned over, and panted, "Sarge, I feel like I'm gonna cry and I want to puke. Is that normal?"

It was perfectly normal. Even though he did everything right and had performed excellently, his adrenaline had still gotten to him.

Are there ways to deal with this? Yes, but it's not easy. Experience is the best system for adrenaline control but it can be hard to survive enough encounters to reap the full benefits. Here are two pieces of advice:

- If you're in a bad situation and you get a warm and happy feeling like you're floating – you're frozen. Recognize the state, and act. Move, punch, scream, or run, but consciously do *something*. Then do something else. That usually breaks you out of the freeze.

- Get used to things going badly. You only have to use unarmed defensive skills when everything else has gone wrong, so take every opportunity to practice recovering from bad positions.

  o   If tournaments scare you, compete.

  o   If someone in your class always beats you, spar with him every day.

  o   Keep going even when you're exhausted.

  o   If you slip and fall, fight from there and insist that your training partners take advantage of the opportunity, just as a threat would.

Concept 10: A threat isn't your training partner

You should see a pattern by now:

▶ Martial arts are relatively safe, fun and healthy.

▶ Fighting is dangerous, unpleasant and potentially crippling.

▶ Martial arts are practiced in a clean environment

▶ Real fighting happens in alleys, bars, and public restrooms.

▶ In martial arts, you know what you're getting into.

▶ In a fight, you might not know if it's a wrestling match or a knife fight until things get slippery.

Here's a big one: you practice martial arts with your friends, people who enjoy spending time with you, who enjoy the art that you enjoy, and who are dedicated to becoming, and helping you become, a better person.

A threat may hate you or despise you with a level of venom that you can barely comprehend. Or the threat may feel no emotion whatsoever, viewing you as nothing more than a source of cash, gratification, or a convenient toy to vent some rage. He might be responding to voices in his head that only he can hear or playing out a scripted fantasy of torture, rape and murder that he has cherished since childhood.

You can't break your partners in training. The ones you spar with tonight will be the ones you spar with next week. *The fact that you're training specifically to break human beings but at the same time you cannot break your training partners is the source of most flaws in martial arts.*

This need to recycle training partners affects what is taught in a martial arts class, and it affects how it's taught. If you have ever been told "We don't do that here, it's too dangerous" or "that's not allowed in a tournament" take a good hard look at why. If you fight non-contact or you hit with contact but only to relatively safe targets, you have been *practicing to miss*. It becomes a habit and, under stress, you will miss just as you have trained to do.

Serious competitive martial artists have stated that just because they don't practice a technique doesn't mean they can't do it. Wrestlers have said that just because they don't practice eye gouging doesn't mean they can't do it. In theory, it's a pretty good argument. What actually happens, however, is that these fighters don't even *think* of using the illegal techniques because they fight the way they have trained. Then, when a threat uses a technique that the martial artist knows as an illegal one, he freezes for a second to reorient. I have actually seen officers getting their asses kicked while looking around for a referee. You fight the way you train and the more intense the training the deeper the habits are ingrained.

That it's hard to train not to injure friends is one half of the problem. The other half is that because of the context of the conflict, threats don't react like training partners.

Most criminals have never been taught to flow with a joint lock or respond in the specific way that you need to make your favorite combination work. Threats who are emotionally disturbed, drunk, drugged, or angry, might not feel pain and won't react to it as your training partners do. Threats have a tendency to flail fast and hard in a continuous jerky action as opposed to those smooth, trained responses you practiced against.

Real threats try to get close to either blitz or sucker-punch; they don't face off at the critical distance line. They don't play the skill and timing game of feint and counter attack. They aren't trying to win; they are trying to hurt you. Threats haven't been taught that a broken nose is a fight-ender.

Look at your training and ask yourself:

- Can I do this if my partner goes full speed?

- Can I do this under the pressure of a flurry of attacks?

- Will it work against a weapon?

- Can I still do it if I can't see clearly?

- Does it take more space than I am likely to have?

- Do real criminals attack the way my partner does in this drill?

- Would it work on me if I were very angry?

In the book "Battle Ready" General Anthony Zinni noted that the lessons he had learned in the jungles of Vietnam didn't help in the Highlands or the rice paddies. Think about that. If the skills of war fighting in a jungle don't help in mountains, swamps or cities, be very careful in presuming that the skills of the ring will help in the chaos of a riot. It's not just that the dojo isn't like the street.

The street isn't always like the street.

Sergeant Rory A. Miller is a corrections officer and tactical team leader for a 2,000 bed jail system. He has studied martial arts since 1981 and worked with inmates since 1991.

At this writing, Rory has participated in over 300 unarmed violent encounters against lone convicts and groups; inmates with and without weapons; inmates on PCP, methamphetamine, and other drugs; and inmates in full-excited delirium.

He teaches and designs such classes as Use of Force, Defensive Tactics and Confrontational Simulation for his agency and, privately, he teaches Sosuishitsu-ryu jujutsu, a Tokugawa era system of close combat. Sergeant Miller has taught seminars around the country.

Rory does his thinking aloud at www.chirontraining.blogspot.com

Many thanks to Luke Heckathorn for posing and to Kamila Z. Miller for her excellent photography.

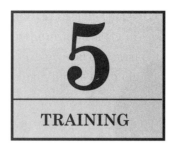

TRAINING

20 Ways to Train and Fight Wounded

By Loren W. Christensen

Here are some bumper stickers on preparedness:

"Confidence comes from being prepared." John Wooden

"If you fail to plan, plan to fail." Anonymous

"Spectacular achievement is always preceded by spectacular preparation." Robert Schuller

As hard training martial artists we are in constant preparation for a self-defense event. We stretch, lift weights, kick, punch, and thrash around on the mats. Our ever-present thought is to be prepared for that moment with well-honed techniques, a sharp and alert mind, and a body that is strong, fast, and healthy. Our mind-set is all about the positive: strong punches, powerful kicks, and incredible speed. But what if some of that were removed by virtue of an injury? A broken elbow not only takes that arm out of the equation, but it saps

83

the entire body of strength, speed and, for some, the will to fight.

Has a fellow student ever blocked your foot so hard that it bent your little toe way back to where it isn't supposed to go, say, on top of your foot? Or maybe you did it yourself kicking a bag. How about your little finger? Ever had it crumpled from someone's heavy-duty block or kick? A little toe and a little finger are tiny body parts with relatively fewer nerve endings than, say, an elbow or knee. Still, injure those little guys and you're off to the sidelines yelping for a warm hug. You don't even want to train anymore tonight, and you're likely to miss a few classes.

A doctor would tell you that that is a wise decision. Give it time to heal, he would advise. Apply some ice, keep the injury elevated, pop some ibuprophen, hit the sofa, and channel surf. While this is excellent advice for your physical injury, it can be argued that it's not so good for your mind. This is because your mind takes this advice and creates an equation. Jammed finger = sofa and TV. Tweaked knee = sofa and TV. Both injuries at the same time = sofa, TV, an adult beverage, and a phone call to mother.

The reason this mindset is arguably a bad thing is that it conditions your thinking to stop fighting, to stop training, to stop everything until you feel better. That works in training, but not on the street. The assailant isn't going to stop thumping on you because you're hurt. That is what he wants. That is his goal. He is going to smell blood and go nuts on you while you're tapping the time-out signal.

Reprogram your mind

Now I'm not saying that you should ignore your injuries. That is never wise and it can come back to bite you in the bee-hind. Take care of your injuries so that they don't become bigger ones that will haunt you years later.

What I am saying is that it's important to train around your injuries to develop a mindset that though you have a broken wrist or a trashed knee cap, you can train and, therefore, you can fight. You might have to hop on one leg or hold your injured arm behind you, but you can, in some way, still hit.

Make a training plan

Whenever I've gotten injured, the first thing that passes through my mind is to ask, how do I train now? Okay, that's not the first thing I think. First I mimic Olympic skater Nancy Kerrigan when she got her knee struck with a baton by an assailant, and I cry out, "Why? Why? Why?" Then I ask myself how I can train.

As I write this it's been about a month since I bent my left big toe back when practicing front kicks on the heavy bag. First it throbbed, then it swelled, and then it turned black. This was especially annoying because I had been making some good gains on the bag. But I swallowed my disappointment and immediately set about planning how I was going to train for the few weeks it would likely take to heal. I had just bought a set of step risers so I decided I would work on those.

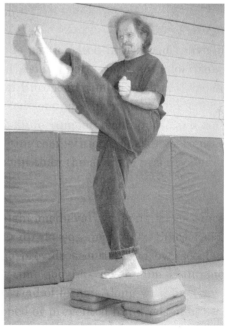

Three times a week I'd step up on the riser, execute a front kick in the air, step down and then repeat.

The first week I couldn't do a fast snapping kick with my injured foot because it hurt too much. So I just did slow kicks to emphasize the kicking muscles. Then after a few days when it felt better and I could kick faster with it, I began pushing to increase the number of reps per minute and the number of minutes per session.

My plan worked great. Over the past month I've progressively increased my time on the step, my stepping speed, the number of reps, and my kicking speed. While I'm not getting the experience of kicking a solid bag, I've improved my cardiovascular system, the muscles around my knees from the step-up action (a sort of mini squat), the larger leg muscles involved in the front kick, and I've entertained my dog. Sometimes I hold him while I'm stepping for added weight resistance and because he thinks it's fun.

While I still front kick the heavy bag with my good leg and do other types of kicks on the bag with both legs that don't impact my trashed toe, I'm coming out of this injury stronger than I was before. Once I'm able to front kick the bag again with my healed foot, it will take only a few workouts to get back into the feel of kicking something.

I've written before on the subject of training around an injury to come out of it stronger, so I'll just mention it briefly in bullet form on the next page.

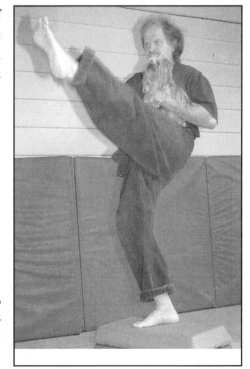

Oh all right! So
he's not that
much resistance.

- When you injure any part of your hand or arm:

  o hold it behind your back and work your drills and sparring as usual.

  o train more on your kicks.

  o concentrate on increasing the strength and speed of your "good" arm.

  o focus on building strength and power in your legs with resistance training.

  o practice sprints to develop explosive speed.

- When you injure any part of your foot or leg:

  o practice kicking and punching reps to understand how the injury affects your balance.

  o if you can't stand on your injured leg or foot, practice your kicks while sitting in a chair (check out *Solo Training DVD* published by YMAA Publication Center for chair kicking exercises). You might be able to practice kicks, even slow ones, with your injured limb.

  o practice all your techniques - kicks, hand, elbow, whatever – while sitting and lying on the floor.

  o if you can support your weight on your injured limb, work your drills and sparring as you usually do.

  o double your training time with your good leg. Some fighters say they don't want one leg better than the other. Why the heck not? If you don't train your good leg while the injured one heals, you come out of your injury with two legs in bad shape. Train so you have a powerful kicking leg should you have to defend yourself during your recuperation period. Then when the other leg heals, work to bring it up to par with your much improved good one.

  o emphasize arm techniques with a goal of increasing their speed, accuracy, power, and explosiveness.

•When you injure your back or neck.

o   Each back and neck injury is different, so you have to experiment to see what hurts it and what might cause further injury. Whatever you *can* do, work that. I've had back injuries that were so severe that all I could do were a few dumbbell curls with one arm while lying on the floor in a strange-looking posture. By the time I recovered from the back injury and could train again that one arm was pretty darn strong.

I could go on listing every possible injury but you get the idea. When you get hurt go ahead, and cry, "Why me? Why me? Why me?" and then go about figuring out what you can do and how you can progress in some way.

No handicap for this guy

One of the many characters I ran across walking a beat on skid row as a cop in Portland, Oregon was a grizzled old timer named Lefty. He told me once that he didn't know if he was given the nickname because he was missing his left leg all the way to his hip or because he only had a right one. Either way, Lefty took both his name and his handicap in stride. He had long since adapted to his prosthetic leg (the vintage pink-colored wood type) and except for a slight limp, he still had a lot of giddy-up in his get-a-long.

One night, a couple of officers came around a corner to find Lefty engaged in a serious fight with a man. Just prior to the officers showing up, both combatants had crashed to the sidewalk. At one point, Lefty had removed his prosthetic limb and was beating the other guy all over his head and body with it, sort of like Sampson did to the army of Philistines with that jawbone.

And like Sampson, he was winning.

So if Lefty can adapt to being physically challenged, you can, too.

Develop a mindset to fight injured

You've got an injury and you have figured out what you can and can't do. You're ready to keep yourself in a training mode and even grow stronger in another area. To make it even more beneficial, you want to work on a mindset that you're able to defend yourself given your incapacitation. One that knows that you can fight and you can fight well. A mindset that is a synergism of accepting your injury, determining a course of action, turning your plan into action, and training with a powerful sense of combat.

Let's make your injury a wrist hyperextension. Since it has swollen to the size of a Volkswagen and the slightest movement with that arm makes your brain hurt, you're forced to give into the reality that you have to let it rest and heal. You've wrapped it or maybe it's even in a sling. But you're going to train anyway. If you can, put your arm behind your back and hook your thumb in your belt. If that hurts too much, move it off to your side as far as you can. You're now good to go.

Bag work

You can certainly practice punching the air with your good arm, and you should for a set of 10 reps to check your body alignment and balance now that you're functioning mostly on only one side. However, only by hitting a heavy bag or a mannequin-style bag will you get a true sense of what it feels like to hit someone with your arm held protectively behind your back.

You don't have to do anything special as far as your bag routine is concerned. In fact, one could argue that it's best to do your regular workout because it's already in your mind. Your purpose now, however, is to execute your jabs, crosses, hooks and backfists with only your good arm, while determining how it feels to you physically. As you discovered when punching and kicking the air, it's surprising how much both arms are involved in your balance, speed, and power. With one arm out of commission, you have to adjust and compensate when hammering the bag.

Your style

Can you keep your same style of fighting or do you have to change it a little?

Will you hold your injured arm side forward or your good arm?

If you normally punch the bag with one arm and hold your other fist near the side of your head (which you should), what are you going to do now that you don't have that arm available to you?

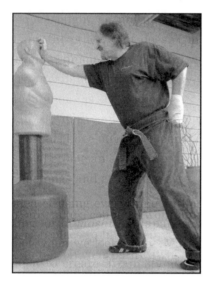

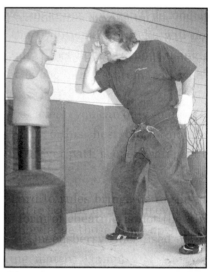

Use the arm you just hit with?

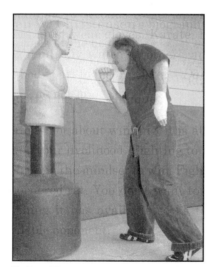

Bob and weave out of range?

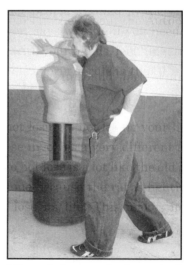

Hit and then push through the bag as if to run past the threat?

These are all good options but you won't know which is best for you until you train with them. You might just find that they are all good and that it just depends on the situation you conjure in your mind.

Defense tactics

How are you going to block? Yes, you can block with your good hand and arm, but what if a kick or punch suddenly comes in on the side of the injured arm?

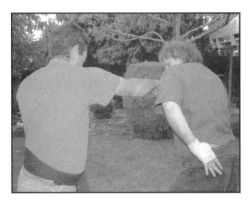 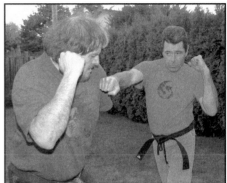

Can you deflect a punch with your shoulder?

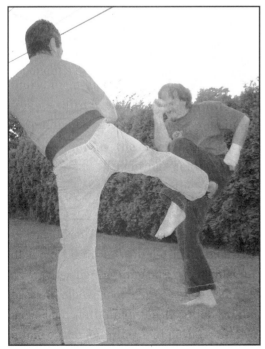

Can you block a kick with your leg?

91

Grappling

I can't begin to count the number of times I had to grapple with resisting suspects when I had but one healthy arm. There were periods I had so many martial arts injuries that I was afraid the PD would try to stifle my training. So I'd drag by crumpled toes, broken fingers and sprained wrists to work, and hide them from my bosses. When I got into a scuffle out in the street, I'd hold my bad arm behind me and get real creative when it came to grappling.

Armbar takedown

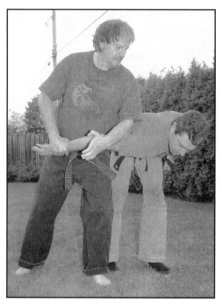 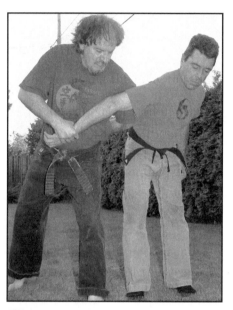

The straight armbar is usually done by gripping the attacker's wrist and applying pressure an inch or so above his elbow.

With one arm out of play, grab his wrist as before and press your upper arm just above his elbow.

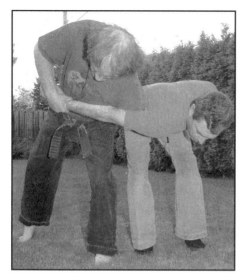

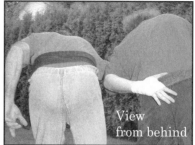

Hold his wrist in place as you turn your upper body slightly to the outside to press the arm down and ultimately take him to the ground.

Wrist twist takedown

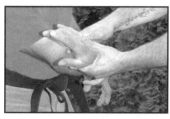

This wrist twist is usually done with two hands.

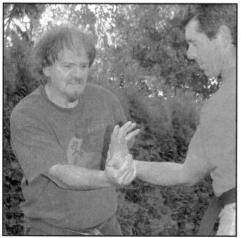

With one arm out of play, twist his hand with one hand.

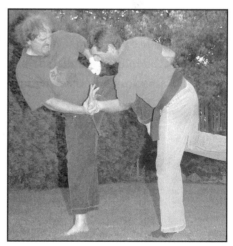

When his weight shifts to his outside leg help him the rest of the way with a knee ram to his midsection.

Hit to help upset his balance

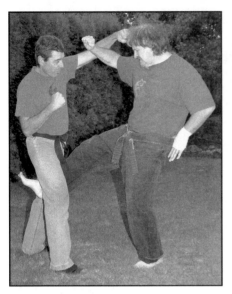

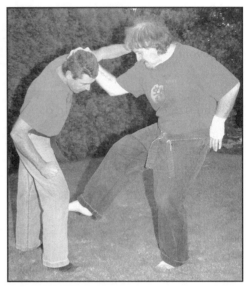

Block his haymaker and simultaneously slam your shin up into his groin.

Grab a wad of hair or cup your hand behind his head...

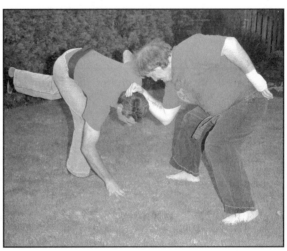

...then jerk your elbow downward to take him to the ground.

More on mindset

I once separated a shoulder fighting an enraged man who had just stabbed another man in the temple with an ice pick. As my adrenaline began to subside after the guy was lying in the backseat of the police car, I realized I couldn't move my left arm. Then I realized it was hurting more and more every passing second. By the time I got back to the station, I was in agony.

Making the pain even more intense was that not only did the injury happen five minutes before my shift ended, the next day I was to defend my title in forms at the Northwest Nationals. No way was that going to happen; no way was I even going to leave my sofa.

After several weeks of physical therapy, my arm still ached but I could move it fairly well. So I asked my physical therapist if he thought I would be able to compete in another tournament three weeks away. He was a martial artist himself and understood. He said that I could, but it would likely set my recovery back a few weeks. If that was okay with me, he said it was okay with him. I thought about it for a couple days and then after deciding I would do it, I changed my mind. No plastic trophy was worth going through the pain and therapy again. However, for a day or so I at least *knew* I could have done it. It would hurt but I knew the adrenaline rush of competition would block the pain and give me the "juice" I needed to perform.

On one occasion during my recuperation, I experienced that same decisiveness when I thought I'd have to deal physically with a violent guy on my commuter train. He had knocked a few people around and was heading my way down the aisle. My mind immediately flashed: *threat...defense...bad arm...I can do it... I will do it...his butt is grass and I'm the lawnmower.*

Overconfidence? Maybe, maybe not. The situation ended without violence so I'll never know. Now, I might not have made the best showing with that bad arm, but the guy would have known he was up against someone nicknamed "Lefty" who was no pushover. A guy who had trained around his injury and who had learned what he could and couldn't do.

And what he could do, he had made strong.

Be smart

Understand that I'm not saying to ignore your injuries. Recognize them as a serious event in your training life and know that not taking care of them properly will only delay your healing and possible cause greater injury. Here are some steps to take when hurt.

- Any severe and long-lasting pain needs to be examined by a doctor.

- Heed the doctor's advice as to what is best to facilitate healing.

- Understand the limitations your injury places on you and don't go beyond those boundaries.

- When something hurts it, don't do that thing anymore.

- Tell your teacher about your injury so that he doesn't ask you to do things to hurt it. If he ignores your injury and pushes you to a place where you might hurt it more, stop training. If he ridicules your actions, you need to seriously consider quitting the school and looking elsewhere.

- Don't let comments from other students make you do something that might hurt you further.

Remember these points:

- Understand your injury and know what you can and cannot do.

- Figure out how to train around it, which means using the healthy parts of your body, not the damaged part.

- Train so that you come out of the injury physically stronger in an area that doesn't involve the injured one, and so that you have the confidence, through self-knowledge, that you can still defend yourself.

---

*L*oren W. Christensen's biography appears in the "About the Author" page at the back of the book. Thanks to Mark Whited for posing and to Lisa Christensen for her fine photography.

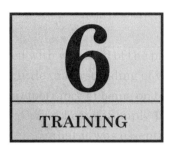

25 Ways to Build Hitting Power Using the Makiwara

By Lawrence Kane

The only time I've been sucker-punched was at a college fraternity party in 1985. He was a 22-year-old, 310-pound Samoan football player, a guy twice my weight and strong as an ox. Although his blow caught me along the side of my jaw, knocking me to the ground, I was back on my feet doing my best Bruce Lee imitation seconds later.

While I ultimately lost, I received only a sore jaw and a bloody nose. My opponent, who barely flinched under my best shot, wasn't seriously injured either. In retrospect, the two of us thumping on each other to no effect was funny. By the time the altercation was over, we held a grudging respect for each other's ability to take a punch; later on, we even became friends after a fashion. We did not realize it at that time, but despite his strength and my agility neither of us could throw a decent punch.

The hardest I've ever been hit happened recently in a karate class when a 57-year-old, 165-pound Japanese *Naha-te* practitioner nearly broke my leg blocking my kick with his arm. He was demonstrating a fighting application (*kata bunkai*) at the time and even pulled his blow, yet I hobbled around without putting my full weight on my right leg for a couple of days afterward. The bruises lasted over a month.

The important lesson from this is that size and strength alone mean little in a fight if you do not know how to punch or kick correctly. Fighters who rely on external power become weaker as they age, but martial artists who use internal power and focused technique become stronger as they gain more knowledge and skill. With superior technique, age matters not.

While the football player used his enormous arm strength to thump me, his "push punch" only knocked me down, though he hit me numerous times. The karate master, on the other hand, used superior technique to create shock, transmitting the full weight of his body and all his energy with his blow. One punch from him was more effective than a dozen from a younger, stronger man. And he wasn't even trying to hit hard! This is a good example of the Japanese concept of *ikken hissatsu* which, roughly translated, means "one blow, one kill," the ability to deliver fight-ending power with every punch.

Ikken hissatsu

The traditional martial arts were developed long before the advent of modern medicine. In those days almost any damage suffered in a fight could ultimately prove fatal via incapacitation, infection, or other collateral impact. Since the shorter duration of the fight the less likelihood of injury to the practitioner, the ancient masters who developed these arts were very concerned about ending fights quickly and decisively. If they could end a confrontation with a single blow so much the better.

Even today, if you lose a fight on the street there is no guarantee that you will walk away without permanent injury, or that you will even walk away at all. If lucky, you might get to resolve your differences over a beer and a game of pool afterward as I did with the football player at the frat party. If unlucky, your adversary might not stop once he has beaten you down. Even if he lets you live, you might still be raped, robbed, or violated in other unpleasant ways before he finishes with you.

If you face off against a skilled street attacker, your opportunities to successfully land a blow are limited. Therefore, you need to make each one count. The first person who lands a solid blow to a vital area earns a huge advantage even if it doesn't end the fight right away. Blocks can also be fight ending or fight ameliorating if applied properly (see Chapter 11 "Shock Blocks"). I have witnessed several instances where a skilled martial artist broke or dislocated his attacker's arm using a traditional block, ending the confrontation without the need to throw an offensive blow. It finished the fight and also kept the practitioner out of jail.

Power test

Do you have the skill to generate fight-stopping power? Short of trying out your martial prowess in a street brawl there are ways to find out. One method is to tape a couple of thick phone books together and have a partner hold them against his chest. Punch the phone books. If your partner feels a pushing sensation or surface pressure, you are using external power and/or poor body alignment. Your *kime* (focus/penetration) is weak. If he feels shock deep within his chest, you are striking correctly.

A good karate punch delivered in the ikken hissatsu method should rock just about anyone's world, even through two large phone books. Using the whole body to focus internal power rather than "separating" the body in a manner that forces reliance on brute muscle strength is a key aspiration of many martial styles. These punches create instantaneous explosive force, delivering hydrostatic shock deep within the body that devastates an adversary. Unfortunately, if you are anything like me, it takes years of diligent practice to get to the point of being able to do that, let alone to do it consistently.

The trick to developing ikken hissatsu is to work on your kime, delivering techniques with proper body alignment, quickness, and power so that you transmit the full force of your body and all your energy at the moment of impact.

The time-honored means of perfecting this ability is through makiwara training.

Gichin Funakoshi, founder of Shotokan karate, wrote, "The most popular way of training with the *seiken* (fore fist or traditional karate punch) is to make use of a makiwara, a thick post covered with rice straw. The makiwara also may be used in strengthening the *shuto* (sword hand), the elbows, and the knees. I think I am in no way exaggerating when I say that practice with the makiwara is the keystone in creating strong weapons."

What is a makiwara?

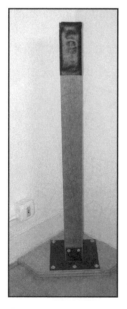

Makiwara means "striking post." Maki translates to "roll up" or "coil" while wara means "straw." The traditional karate striking post was a board wrapped with a straw coil on one end and the other end buried in the ground. For clarity, this is completely different than the rolled straw targets of the same name used by kyudo archers. For those of you who practice Korean martial arts the terminology used there is *dallyon joo*, which translates as "forging post." Dallyon joo is constructed similarly and used in the same manner as a makiwara. There is no traditional Chinese equivalent, though the wooden dummy (*muk yang jong*) plays much the same role in some types of kung fu training.

There are two major styles of makiwara—*tachi* (standing) and *age* (hanging). The tachi-makiwara is a standing post buried in the ground or affixed to a bracket on the floor. It is most often made from a flat, flexible board though you may occasionally find one built from a split circular pole with a rubber pad set inside it and a straw wrap on the outside. Either way, the top is padded, traditionally with rice straw, though today it's often covered with leather or canvas, and a thin layer of closed-cell foam. The flat board version is only struck from the front while the thick pole can be attacked from all sides.

The age-makiwara is a smaller padded board that is suspended from a rope similar to a boxer's speed bag. Age-makiwara are portable, though they are primarily used for kicks and elbow strikes.

You can occasionally find a box-like makiwara designed to be affixed to a wall too, though that style is not traditional and frequently damages the wall behind it when struck repeatedly with force. Another form of makiwara is called a *tou*. It is a bundle of cane or bamboo stalks tied together with a straw rope, and used for finger strikes. Striking a regular makiwara with your finger tips is dangerous and should not be done.

Makiwara helps you develop powerful technique while forging a strong fighting spirit, two fundamental aspects of surviving a street fight.

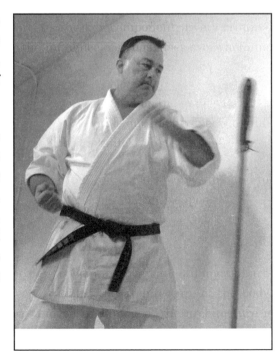

You can practice hand techniques (te waza), leg techniques (ashi waza), receiving or blocking techniques (uke waza), conditioning exercises (tanren), stances (kime, dachi), and moving/shifting techniques (tae sabaki waza). It can even be used for some weapons forms.

> Goju Ryu karate legend Morio Higaonna wrote, "Makiwara training is essential because it develops your technique, your kime. Through diligent practice on the makiwara you will learn how to transmit your full bodily force at the exact moment of impact, from your hand, into an object. Another important benefit is that such practice will forge a strong spirit."

Is it safe to use a makiwara?

With prudent and proper training, the makiwara is safe to use. Contrary to popular misconception, the main purpose of makiwara training is not to break down your hands and re-build them into lethal club-like weapons via micro-fractures in the knuckles. Few martial artists would willingly participate in an activity that was guaranteed to cause them lifelong challenges performing important tasks central to their existence, like feeding themselves and signing their name. Yet you will find one or more makiwara in nearly every traditional dojo throughout the world. Long-term training on the makiwara may produce unsightly keratinized skin but that is limited to natural padding from calluses. The underlying structure of the hand is unaffected.

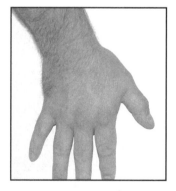

Most people have developed at least a few calluses as a natural defense against prolonged and repeated rubbing and/or pressure on the hands or feet. Many students develop a callus along the middle finger from regular use of a pen or pencil. Similarly, stringed instrument musicians often develop calluses on their fingertips. This skin thickening protects the fingers, allowing extended play without discomfort. If a beginning player practices too long, however, a painful blister may form. The same is true with makiwara work. If you overdo it early in your training you are bound to feel discomfort if not outright pain.

Several studies have been conducted to ascertain the safety of impact training in martial arts. In a 1985 *British Journal of Sports Medicine* report, for example, the study by A. C. Crosby concluded that "long term and routine practice of karate does not appear to predispose to early onset of osteoarthritis or tendonitis in the hands of those studies." A 1970 report by H. J. Larose published in the journal *Medicine and Science in Sports* revealed a comparison of karate master Sosai Masutatsu (Mas) Oyama's hands which were x-rayed in 1955 and again in 1970. Although the founder of Kyokushinkai karate performed daily drills on the makiwara for fifteen years between examinations the report found that, "There was no evidence of any kind of degenerative disease of the bones or joints. The density and size of the bones and joints were normal. There was no evidence of old fractures of any bone. There was no evidence of calcification (new bone formation) of the bones, joints, or soft-tissues."

Reviewing these studies and others, sports medicine guru Keith McCormack concluded that, "Using recognized toughening drills, appropriate to your level of training, correctly executed techniques will not cause damage to your hands." His conclusions were published in the December 1985 issue of *Fighting Arts International*. My personal experience and that of my instructors as well as my students concurs with his findings.

Safety Tips

- Should you injure your knuckles, stop training until they are fully healed. In most cases you may still strike the makiwara with uninjured parts of the hand or foot.

- Do not use the makiwara if you have an open wound. If anyone is cut and bleeds on the makiwara striking pad, clean the affected area with a mixture of bleach and water to reduce the possibility of blood-borne pathogen contamination. While HIV can only survive for a few seconds outside the body, certain contagions such as hepatitis can even be transmitted via dried blood.

- Only train under proper supervision until you have developed a level of expertise that your sensei feels is appropriate to warrant practice on your own.

- Exercise proper form when punching—keep your wrist straight and do not lock your elbow at full extension. Proper body alignment not only increases the power of your technique but also protects against injury.

- Hit only with the appropriate portion of your hand or foot. When performing *seiken tsuki* (fore fist punch) or *tate tsuki* (standing punch), for example, connect with only your first two knuckles (80 percent impact on the first knuckle). Wrist injuries or boxer's fractures (breaking the metacarpal along the top of the hand and/or breaking the knuckle of the little or ring finger) are likely to occur if you hit improperly.

- Do not perform finger strikes or head butts on the makiwara. Either technique is likely to cause injury.

- Start with half-power blows, aiming at the surface of the board. Gradually increase the force you apply over time, shifting your aim further and further through the makiwara. Limit the number of punches you throw with each part of your hand (e.g., knuckles, palm, edge), especially in your first few training sessions. Overtraining can cause injuries that will inhibit your progress as you are forced to wait until they heal.

- Do not let young children use the makiwara. A practitioner's hand should be fully developed before striking any solid surface. Depending on the individual, youths 16 years of age and older should be able to use the makiwara safely under supervision.

- Ensure that the makiwara is properly built and in good repair. There should be no splinters or cracks in the wood. It should retain sufficient flexibility to absorb blows and possess adequate padding. It is better for it to be too flexible than not flexible enough.

Kickboxers can use it, too

Is makiwara training only for traditional karate and taekwondo practitioners? "No," say both Loren Christensen, a teacher of street-oriented martial arts and this book's author and editor, and Wim Demeere, European sanshou champion and veteran muay Thai fighter.

"Although it's typically thought of as a training tool for students of Shotokan, Goju and other Japanese disciplines," Christensen says, "anyone can use it, and should. For sure, a heavy bag or hand pad will let you know when you're hitting incorrectly, but they show you in a relatively nice way. A makiwara is crueler as it sends your tweaked wrist into the pain zone or swells those knuckles you shouldn't be making contact with. When you know of its innate cruelty, it forces you to learn quickly the proper way to hit. In doing so, you develop an understanding of precise body mechanics as your power, focus and accuracy increases rapidly."

I asked Christensen if the makiwara board is applicable for a fighter with a high guard. "Sure," Christensen says. "Why not? A target is a target. The makiwara isn't just for traditionalists who punch primarily from the hip. I hold my hands and arms in a high guard with my fists between my chin and ears, and the position is perfect for makiwara work."

Muay Thai and sanshou expert Wim Demeere agrees. He particularly likes how the makiwara helps to develop pinpoint targeting. "Kickboxers are used to hitting the broad surfaces of heavy bags and kicking shields," Demeere says. "The makiwara offers a much smaller target, which enhances hitting accuracy."

Demeere debunked the myth of static punching. "Many people think you have to stand in front of the makiwara rooted in place as you hit it. Not true. For example, I like to hit it with hook punches. One way to do that is to step to the left diagonally with the lead leg (when doing a right hook), which brings you up alongside the target, and launch a right hook punch, landing it square-on with your knuckles. There's less hip rotation involved to generate power using a drop-step. First the move gets you off line with your assailant and your drop-step helps you land a very powerful hook into his solar plexus or chest plate."

How to use a makiwara

The makiwara can be used to reinforce proper form and to perfect power. There are two primary ways to use it: slow work and impact work. Slow work builds form while impact work perfects power. You can do both simultaneously, of course, but it is a bit easier to explain and less difficult to practice when broken into component parts. Since form is a necessary precursor of power, I'll cover slow work first.

Slow work

A traditional way of practicing proper form in the dojo is via *sanchin shimé* (testing of technique and power). The way it works is that students complete *sanchin kata* (a core form of many martial systems) while an instructor checks concentration, body alignment, movement, breathing, and mechanics of their technique by giving pressure and striking various parts of the student's body. The teacher's slaps and pushes provide essential validation and reinforcement.

Shimé testing helps practitioners focus on parts of the body that are not actively being used so that they do not forget about them, facilitating a practitioner's ability to concentrate on his or her whole body simultaneously. These same principles can be applied using a makiwara in your solo training.

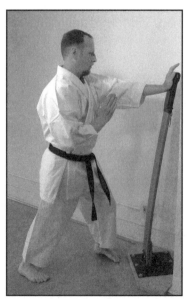

To test the stability of your stance, press against the makiwara with your palm using the progressive resistance as the board bends. In a properly formed *sanchin dachi* (hourglass stance), for example, force should travel through your arm and body downward into your back heel. No matter how far you push the makiwara (and how hard it pushes back), your alignment should not waver. You can test all your stances in this fashion.

Similarly, you can slowly deliver any type of punch, block, or kick and feel the effect of reverse pressure against your body, checking for stance, body alignment, and effective technique. Practice each technique slowly and smoothly, keeping the resistance from spoiling your form. Use abdominal breathing to help focus your power and keep your center of balance low, inhaling through the nose and out the mouth. Check your alignment both at the moment of impact as well as throughout your full natural extension.

Impact work

While slow work develops proper alignment, impact work builds penetrating power. Proper kime requires coordination of mind, body, and breathing, which is a lot more complicated than it sounds, yet it is easily facilitated via the makiwara.

When struck with force, the makiwara provides positive reinforcement when you get it right and painful negative reinforcement when you get it wrong. You get kinesthetic, visual, and auditory feedback.

When struck properly, you can feel the impact, see the board snap back, and hear an explosive cracking noise.

This is not caused by the board breaking but rather by it flexing with alacrity. Strike it improperly, however, and the board will bend back and make a dull thump or creak rather than snapping back with force. It may also hurt your fist and/or wrist to strike improperly (a few improper blows will probably not cause any lasting injury, yet pain does facilitate rapid self-correction).

So if you can feel, see, and hear a good blow but are having difficulty executing one consistently, how do you get it right? Proper alignment is crucial, especially when punching something solid. Individual bones in the fingers and hand cannot withstand much force by themselves, but as a solid integrated unit they are very strong.

- Start with a good, tight fist. Keep your elbow close to the body, aligning the knuckles and wrist.

- For a standard punch, there should be a nice straight line of force starting at the point of impact on your first/second knuckle, traveling through your wrist, up your arm, through your shoulder, and into your body.

o   Not only does striking with the first two knuckles help properly align the force and protect your hand, but it delivers force across a smaller surface area, hence striking with more penetrating power.

- Relax the deltoid muscles in the shoulder, tightening the latissimus and pectoral muscles on impact for best speed and power with a standard punch.

- Align your hand and wrist.

- To create a force path from your hand into your torso, your shoulder should be low and relaxed, not raised or extended.

- With a proper stance and muscle tension, your upper and lower body should become one solid unit.

o   If your body is not integrated, you only hit with the power of your arm.

o   When your spine is straight and your body integrated, you hit with the power of your whole being.

- Do not fully extend and lock your arm, however, as you may damage your elbow joint.

- Tighten all the muscles in your arm but do not lock the elbow.

Fa....jing!!

Fa jing means explosive or vibrating power. It is sort of like a sneeze, a sudden unexpected movement. Speed and relaxation are necessary to achieve fa jing, followed by an instant of tension at the moment of impact. All punches should be performed in this fashion. Once you progress past slow work, never "pull" your punch. If you wish to strike lightly aim for the front edge of the makiwara and punch with full power. If you wish to strike hard, aim through the makiwara. Your point of aim determines the level of impact.

Be sure to practice techniques from static stances as well as when moving toward and away from the makiwara from various angles. Being able to strike while moving is very important in a real fight. You must be able to deliver both offensive and defensive techniques while moving, shifting, and evading an adversary's blows. Try both stepping and shifting movements with each technique, ensuring that you end up in proper range with good posture at the moment of impact. Work on disguising your weight shift then exploding into your target.

No such thing as a "weak side"

Since you never know which blow will ultimately connect in a street fight, you must be able to hit hard and make every blow count with every limb. Morio Higaonna wrote, "If a right-handed student strikes the makiwara 100 times, he should try striking it 200 times with his left hand. Students should always practice two or three times more with their weaker and less developed parts of the body than with those parts which are already well developed." This is sound advice.

Training Tips

- Use a wide variety of techniques, not just punches. Try standing fist (*tate tsuki*), sword hand (*shuto uchi*), palm heel (*shotei uchi*), hammerfist (*tetsui uchi*), backfist (*uraken tsuki*), wrist strike (*koken tsuki*), swing strike (*furi uchi*), elbow strike (*hiji ate*), knee strike (*hiza geri*), front kick (*mae geri*), side kick (*yoko geri*), and so on.

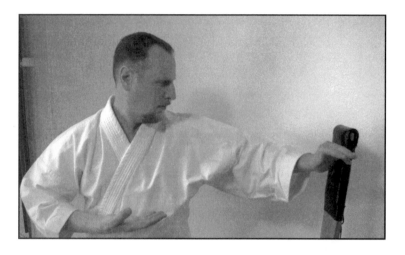

- Practice striking from a variety of stances such as hourglass stance (*sanchin dachi*), sumo stance (*shiko dachi*), front stance (*zenkutsu dachi*), and cat leg stance (*neko ashi dachi*). Use everything you find in your kata, working both from the static stances as well as while moving.

- Maintain your mental focus, performing each blow with perfect form. Ten techniques executed with all your skill are better than a hundred performed haphazardly. Not only are you more likely to become injured with sloppy form, but you will also be reinforcing poor technique. What you do in training will heavily influence what you will do on the street.

- Work both your strong side and your weak side. Unless you are ambidextrous it is a good idea to practice two to three times as many repetitions on your weak side as you do on your dominant side.

- Practice speed and form to create power, relaxing until the moment of impact then tensing the whole body. Pay attention to the sound the impact makes to reinforce proper technique. A solid, well-delivered blow will cause an explosive cracking noise while a brute force push punch will only make a dull thump.

- Be sure you stand close enough to the makiwara to strike it with good form from either hand. In proper range, your *gyaku tsuki* (reverse punch) should be able to bend the makiwara to maximum desired extension without the need to overextend or roll your shoulder forward. This emulates punching through an adversary rather than at him, reducing the likelihood of surface impact without true "killing" power. If you are too far away, power is dissipated at every point where your body is not properly connected such as when you roll your shoulder or bend forward unnaturally.

- Do not telegraph your punches. Each blow should suddenly explode from chamber (or wherever your starting point is) into your target as fast as possible with no warning. Avoid cocking your arm back, taking a sudden breath, tensing your neck, shoulders, or arms, widening your eyes, grinning, grimacing, or making any other inappropriate movement before each blow. If there is a mirror available it will help you notice and eliminate these foibles. If not, you may wish to videotape your training session and analyze the film afterward.

- Strike directly at the target covering the shortest distance possible. Keep your elbow pointed downward and your arm as close to your side as possible (except for furi uchi and similar techniques).

If you have any hip rotation, it should be slightly up/down rather than side to side. While side-to-side hip rotation helps generate external power, it also forces you to realign your body for each follow-on punch. This not only increases the time it takes to strike the target but also telegraphs your blow. Internally powered punches move faster, strike harder, and do not require this extra movement.

111

Modern punching bag vs. makiwara

While the makiwara and heavy bag can both help build stamina and endurance, the makiwara is structurally superior for traditional martial arts training. To begin, it offers progressive resistance like a bow. Unlike a heavy bag, there is no softness or give at initial contact. The harder you strike against it, the harder the makiwara pushes back. This not only facilitates an ability to validate stance integrity and perform other slow work, but also provides superior kinesthetic, visual, and auditory feedback with impact training.

Soft punching bags are good at cushioning your hand and limiting repetitive impact damage yet they do not adequately simulate hitting a real target, often fomenting bad habits. Miscues that you may not even notice on a punching bag can easily lead to hospitalization on the street. Using bag gloves, taping your wrists, or relying on any other supportive device can exacerbate the problem. Even professional boxers have been known to damage themselves in real fights. For example, former heavyweight champion "Iron" Mike Tyson broke his right hand in a street brawl with boxer Mitch Green on August 23, 1988. You need to be able to strike properly with your naked fist, aligning the knuckles, wrist and arm so that you injure your adversary while not hurting yourself.

If you are going to use a punching bag, a Body Opponent Bag (BOB) is preferable to a traditional heavy bag since it provides solid resistance and more closely simulates striking an adversary. A makiwara, on the other hand, is cheaper to build and offers more flexibility and functionality for martial arts training.

Like any other traditional tool, it would have been discarded long before now if it did not work effectively.

Building a makiwara

Flexibility

The makiwara needs to be flexible to operate properly. It is usually better for it to be too flexible than not flexible enough. The flexibility of the board absorbs enough of the impact to eliminate the need for thick padding, so the covering of straw, leather, canvas, foam, or rubber protects the board almost as much as it protects the practitioner's hand. A properly designed tachi-makiwara should be roughly shoulder height as you take a fighting stance (e.g., sanchin dachi).

Wood

Makiwara are traditionally made of *shijiya* wood (Japanese beech wood family). Japanese cypress and Japanese cedar are also common. Ash, white oak, beech, cherry, hickory, and pine can also work. Regardless of what wood you select, it should be as knot-free as you can find with the grain running straight up and down to the greatest extent possible. Quarter-sawn lumber works best because the grain will almost always be tight, straight, and parallel throughout the entire board.

I like to use a 1" x 4" board with a simple leather wrap over the striking surface. Some folks start with a 4" x 4" board and plane it diagonally starting around 1/3 of the way up such that the base is square but the striking area is flat and only about ¾" thick. It is common to affix a thick canvas/foam striking pad to this style of post. A stiffer board is required to support the weight of a heavy striking pad then is necessary with a thin wrap.

If the board is too thin, you get too much whipping motion from the extra weight at the top and not enough resistance for correct action. Whatever thickness you choose, there are two ways to secure the post at the bottom: bury it in the ground or affix it to a floor-mounted bracket.

Buried vs. affixed

If buried, an 8-foot board is frequently used, with roughly 4 to 5 feet sticking out above the ground. I like to dig a hole in the ground, dump in some quick drying concrete, then place the makiwara post inside along with a secondary board behind it that is about a foot taller than the depth of the partially-filled hole. I then fill in the hole with concrete and hold everything in place while it begins to dry. After the concrete has set up but is not completely dry, I gently remove the shorter board. Once the concrete is completely dry, I re-insert a wedge-shaped board to hold the makiwara post firmly in place. The concrete encapsulates the buried portion of the board, protecting it from rotting and allowing it to last several years outdoors. If the makiwara breaks and needs to be replaced, I simply remove the wedge and drop in a new board without damaging the concrete base.

Alternately the makiwara post can be braced with cross-pieces or large rocks and buried directly in the ground. This is arguably more traditional but does not last as long as a concrete base. Pour in some gravel before placing the board in the hole to facilitate proper drainage.

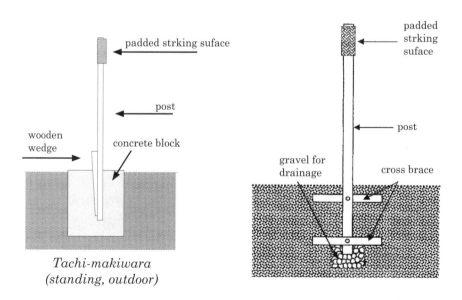

Tachi-makiwara
(standing, outdoor)

Another type of buried makiwara is the pole-style. Like a traditional tachi-makiwara, it either buried in the ground or set in concrete. Unlike the traditional board-style striking post, however, you can strike it from about any angle. This version is used more for weapon forms than empty-hand striking because it is much more rigid.

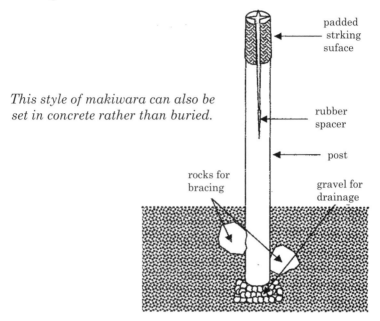

This style of makiwara can also be set in concrete rather than buried.

padded strking suface

rubber spacer

post

rocks for bracing

gravel for drainage

This style can be set in concrete with a wedge rather than buried in the ground with cross bracing.

If you would rather have your makiwara indoors, build a wooden bracket or purchase a metal one to mount your makiwara post to the dojo floor.

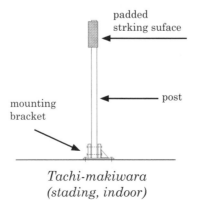

padded strking suface

post

mounting bracket

*Tachi-makiwara
(stading, indoor)*

115

If you don't like putting holes in your floor, mount the bracket to a half sheet of plywood to create a portable stand. Your weight is sufficient to keep the stand from moving while you use the makiwara.

Regardless of how you mount it, any wood used outdoors should be treated with a waterproofing stain or oil. Drop an empty bucket over the striking pad or cover it with plastic when not in use to help it last longer in inclement weather.

Hanging makiwara

To make an age-makiwara, hold two boards together with a rubber pad in between at each end, then wrap with a cord at both ends to secure everything in place. Wrap the outer board with straw rope or leather for striking, and then hang it from a ceiling beam or eyebolt. If you don't have much room, affix a bungee cord to the bottom and secure it to the floor to keep it from swinging around too much during use.

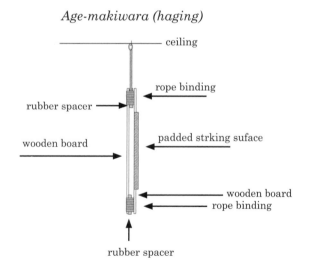

Age-makiwara (haging)

Parting thoughts

A common nickname for a makiwara is the "board of wisdom," since it provides immediate and accurate feedback with each blow, refining technique while forging a warrior spirit as you condition your hands and feet for combat. Makiwara training can strengthen your entire body, perfecting and aligning punches, kicks, blocks, stances, and even movement. It is an ideal way to learn how to deliver fight-stopping blows with focus, power, and penetration.

Disclaimer

Makiwara training can be dangerous if undertaken incorrectly. Use only a properly built makiwara, performing all techniques under the guidance and supervision of a qualified instructor.

---

*L*awrence Kane is the author of *Surviving Armed Assaults* and *Martial Arts Instruction* as well as the coauthor of *The Way of Kata*. He has also published numerous articles about teaching, martial arts, self-defense, and related topics, and is a forum moderator at www.iainabernethy.com, a web site devoted to traditional martial arts and self-protection.

Over the last 30 plus years, Lawrence has participated in a broad range of martial arts, everything from traditional Asian sports such as judo, arnis, kobudo, and karate to recreating medieval European combat with real armor and rattan weapons. He has also completed seminars in modern gun safety, marksmanship, handgun retention, and knife combat techniques, and has participated in slow-fire pistol and pin shooting competitions. These experiences give him a somewhat more diverse viewpoint than the average practitioner of such arts.

As a martial arts instructor, he has taught medieval weapons forms since 1994 and has been teaching Goju Ryu karate classes since 2002. Since 1985, Lawrence has supervised employees who provide security and oversee fan safety during football games. This part-time job has given him a unique opportunity to appreciate violence in a myriad of forms. Along with his crew, he has witnessed, interceded in, and stopped or prevented hundreds of fights, experiencing all manner of aggressive behaviors as well as the escalation process that invariably precedes them. He also works closely with law enforcement officers assigned to the stadium and has had ample opportunities to examine their crowd control tactics and procedures. He likes to think of it as getting paid to watch football... at least until somebody pulls a knife or starts a riot.

To pay the bills, Lawrence works for a large aerospace company where he is responsible for sourcing strategy and benchmarking activities in Information Technology. In other words, he gets to play with billions of dollars of other people's money and make really important decisions.

Lawrence can be contacted via e-mail at lakane@ix.netcom.com.

Thanks to Kris Wilder for his work as a model and as a photographer.

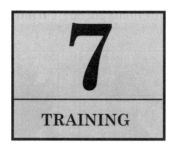

10 Ways to a Stronger Punch

By Kris Wilder

"Reality is that which, when you stop believing in it, doesn't go away."
- writer Philip K. Dick

Our understanding of violence today is vastly different than it was in ancient times. Think about the time and place karate comes from and how that contrasts with today's world. Technological advances have changed drastically the way we view violence. For example, in a typical metropolitan area a police officer or firefighter is only moments away. DNA testing links criminals to crime scenes that are decades old, street lights illuminate your path home, and sophisticated locks secure your home and car. Cell phones and Global Positioning Systems communications allow for pinpoint accuracy in finding a location. Torn ligaments are mended with arthroscopic surgery, broken bones are set and healed in ultra-light casts, and antibiotics help cuts heal faster. Two hundred years ago on Okinawa, a small island in the Pacific, none of these things existed.

In today's world, we live under the illusion that we're safe – our modernity and our superior knowledge means we won't be called to defend ourselves because we are so unlikely to be personally attacked. Television and films have further served to distort reality by presenting over-the-top examples of violence and unreal responses and outcomes, as well as desensitizing us to its true nature. Violence is "out there" and it happens to other people. The truth is that real violence, just like Philip K. Dick says, "...doesn't go away." It just looks a lot different that most people think.

The karate-ka of the past knew what violence was in a very real sense and they understood that a violent act changed everybody involved, and that fighting was a serious affair. They passed that knowledge on in their forms to relatives and friends.

Almost every martial art has forms, patterns, or kata that serve as "textbooks" of how to fight. But there is a deep undercurrent to fighting at the structural level that is beyond technique. Specifically housed within a kata is a deeper knowledge regarding preparation of the body for fighting, preparation which is often overlooked. For example, part of an overarching strategy for the karate-ka is to set his body to deliver a bone-jarring blow to an opponent but to not allow the opponent's strikes to penetrate his.

To better understand the origins and goals of karate techniques, a solid understanding of history as well as attitudes and definitions surrounding violence is helpful in bringing forward the old way of fighting into today's world.

Three roles of violence

In the modern world, violence falls into the role of the citizen, the role of the police, and the role of the military. These roles have not changed much over history, only different combinations, and different mixtures.

The citizen

The citizen's role regarding violence is to escape, which, while sounding cowardly is frankly the best option. This is because "Joe Average" citizen doesn't train to fight or engage in physical violence, while the person who has selected Joe Average for an act of violence has most likely been violent in the past and believes that Joe is an easy mark. Choosing him stacks the odds in favor of the attacker. The best solution for Joe Average is to separate from the threat before the threat separates him from his senses, money, or his life.

The police officer

The police role is to stop violent activity. Officers are trained to do the opposite of the citizen: They move toward the violence, take charge, and make it end. This role of stopping violence makes lethal force the last in line of many other options. Watch any cop show and you will see this progression occur: words, words, words, implied force, force, injury, and finally, lethal force.

The military

The military's role is to kill the enemy combatant and break their things. The military prefers to do this as fast as possible, as the longer they are engaged the more that can go wrong. The more that goes wrong in battle the higher the possibility of injury or death to members of one's own military.

Assessing the situation

Making an accurate and instant assessment of your attacker's capability and intentions is the most important evaluation you can make. Understanding the roles of the players before anything happens is vital.

Karate makes a military decision in a civilian atmosphere. At its very core karate is about stopping the other guy as fast as possible. Traditional karate, from a physical standpoint, is a tendon-snapping, bone-breaking, high-risk activity not to be entered into lightly as everybody's life will be different once it is over.

Two hundred years ago a broken bone meant you didn't work, and there was no workers' compensation or unemployment. A torn ligament meant you might not be able to contribute to the family, or pull your own weight. An infection from a compound fracture, where the bone actually breaks through the skin, could well mean death.

Living on a small island in the Pacific Ocean 200 hundred years ago meant you didn't enter into fighting lightly; when you did engage, it was a serious affair. Your technique needed to be good, of course, but more important the structural integrity of your technique had to be rock solid. In addition, your combat strategy, distinctly different from policing and civilian strategies had to make sense. Today, as in ancient times, honing your strategy and solidifying your architecture are the keys to increasing your odds of success in a violent encounter.

Below is a discussion of a variety of time-tested techniques to employ when faced with violence. It is important to note that even though some of the techniques might be mutually exclusive, meaning you can't do one if you are doing the other, that doesn't mean the traditional karateka will not use whatever technique they need to win. Only a fool fights without using every resource available to them. To say, "That is not in my system, so I won't use that technique." is sheer idiocy.

Cheating

The idea of using everything without regard to rules brings us to the idea of cheating, or *damashu* in Japanese. This form of cheating is not the kind we think of when we look at the Marquess of Queensberry rules used in boxing. Designed to create a fair stand-up boxing match, examples of Marquess of Queensberry these rules include no wrestling, 3-minute rounds, when a fighter falls he has 10 seconds to get up, no other people allowed in the ring, and fighters must wear gloves. Karate, however, says wrestle if you need to, end the fight quickly, watch for others, and hit with your hands, feet, fingers or any other body part to insure victory. *Damashu* is a form of rule in that it is no rule – cheat, do not lose.

Karate is not about winning; it is about not losing – not losing your life, your limb, or your livelihood. Fighting to not lose involves a very different attitude than having the mindset to win. Fighting to not lose is a lot like the old analogy of a cornered rat. You don't want to fight one because the rat is fighting with everything it has available so as to not lose its life. This makes it a very formidable opponent.

Even Sun Tzu says you need to leave an enemy a means of escape.

Sun Tzu on cornered armies

"Soldiers placed in dire situations lose their sense of fear. If there is no place of safety, they will stand firm. If there is no help available to them, they will fight hard."

~ *The Art of War*

The Strategy of body mechanics

Strategy is what is done in preparation to go to battle while tactics are what are done on the battlefield. Consider taekwondo: the art's strategy is to use more kicking techniques than hand techniques; using a crescent and ax kick combination would be an example of a tactic. Strategies of the Okinawa school would include a posture where the body is locked down, with the torso and abdomen together in a solid piece that is rooted to the ground, using shorter strikes with more hands than kicking, and using aggressive movement into the opponent's space and breaking their balance.

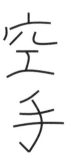

Important point: Being able to withstand a blow is the flip side of being able to generate a powerful strike. One begets the other – they are not separate activities when it comes to fighting. Taking and giving blows originate from the same platform; the same architecture is used.

*K*arate

Delivering bone-jarring impact

If you have ever stepped off a curb unexpectedly or missed a step that you thought was there, you felt the bone-jarring, teeth-rattling transfer of energy through your body. This sensation is the one that traditional karate attempts to drive into body of the aggressor when striking.

Here are some of the cornerstones to developing the bone-jarring energy transfer that is at the very core of all karate techniques, including strikes, aggressive defense, throws, locks and others.

The preparation of the body   It has been said by many martial arts instructors through the ages that you must be like a tree in generating martial power. Frankly, there is not a more apt or easy to understand explanation than this analogy, so we will use it to help us in preparing the body to strike and generate power.

The roots equal the feet   Poor roots in a tree means that a strong storm might blow the tree over. Poor footing means that you as a fighter will wind up on the ground. In karate, going to the ground is a very bad thing. It is essential to be secure in your footing and, therefore, the shoes you choose to wear are the beginning of this process.

Bad shoes:

- Cowboy boots have heels that keep you off the ground and roll you forward onto the balls of your feet. This is bad for generating power.

- Leather soles, like the ones on many dress shoes, can be slick enough without adding a splash of water from a barroom urinal or blood on the floor.

Bottom line: heels and slick soles are poor conductors of energy.

Good shoes:

- Any footwear that has a low heel and a sole with good traction.

Linking to the ground Placing the foot on the ground and linking with the ground is the first fundamental element of generating power. The sensation is that of being stuck in shallow mud, as if the wet earth had rolled up around the edges of the foot. The heels of your feet remain planted in the earth. Do not mistake this for being heavy or lethargic in your foot movement, because moving quickly, such as getting out of the way of a strike is always preferable to being struck.

Important point: When striking, you are linked to the ground for that brief instant your blow contacts with the opponent. The following illustrations demonstrate the difference between being linked to the ground with the entire foot down, and lifting the heel of the foot, unlinking the body from the ground.

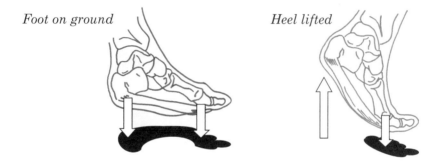

Foot on ground *Heel lifted*

The Knees

In traditional karate the knees oftentimes have the appearance of being locked, even hyperextended. In fact, the femur and the tibia are aligned, stacked on top of one another, creating a straight line of power to the ground.

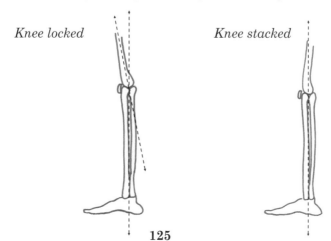

Knee locked *Knee stacked*

Stacking, and not locking, allows for a better generation of power and yet permits swift movement when mobility is required. It also keeps the opponent from seeing the motion of the unlocking of the knee reverberate throughout the body prior to a body shift. This reverberation, or hitch, in preparation to shifting or striking, tips off the opponent that you are preparing to move. Try this test:

Stand in front of a friend close enough to touch his chest when you extend your hand.

- Ask him to slap your hand down as you attempt to touch him on the chest.

- Try it a couple of times to see the results.

- Now, without saying anything to tip him off, simply twitch the shoulder of your striking hand ever so slightly and watch the reaction.

The point here is that your opponent can see even the slightest movement you make and he reacts quickly to the visual cues. But when there are no clues, no tells, and no tips, you suddenly become fast.

The puff vs. the bow

The next time you see a fight, watch for the bowing of the back or the puffing up of the chest. These indicate two very different things that are worth noticing.

Puffing up the chest is a display, a threat. It is like a chicken ruffling up its feathers to look bigger or a gorilla ripping grass from the ground and beating its chest. The Puff says, "I am dangerous! Look out! Run away! You don't want any of this!" The Puff always starts at a safe distance.

The bow, on the other hand, indicates an actual preparation to fight, and is done just prior to or during the closing of distance. The bowing of the back and the dropping of the chin is as real as you get when it comes to preparing the body for violence. While the puff is all show, the bow is all go. The puff is about proving something; the bow is about doing something.

The Spine

The spine is designed to absorb the bumps of the day. When you compress and expand, sway from side to side, and twist left and right, your spine is always at work keeping you balanced and serving as the body's main structural support, the core of the torso and abdomen.

Locking the spine allows for the transference of power from the ground to the opponent through the spine, and does so in a manner that, when executed correctly, transfers as much kinetic energy as possible into the body of the opponent.

Five points of the spine need to be set to transfer kinetic energy from the ground through the body to the opponent: The Coccyx, Lumbar 5, Thorax 11, Cervical 7, and Cervical 1. The proper alignment of these five points in the spine is essential to providing the power that is often seen in the bowing of the back of a skilled fighter regardless of discipline. Here is a brief outline of this technique:

1. Rotate the coccyx underneath the sacrum.

2. Push Lumbar #5 backward away from the abdomen.

3. Pull Thorax #11 inward toward the solar plexus.

4. Pull Cervical #7 in line on top of Thorax #11.

5. Pull Cervical #1 backward and over the top of Cervical #7.

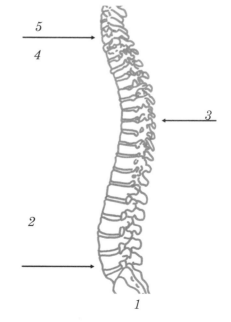

Shoulders

Under stress, the human body tends to lift the shoulders. At the first dump of adrenaline the shoulders lift, the head drops and the hands move in front of the body in a defensive position. This shoulder lift is counter to what old-school karate tells you to do. No form or kata explicitly tells you to lift your shoulder up to your ears. In fact, traditional karate teaches to drop the shoulders to avoid allowing the shoulder to move up or down or forward and backward.

The shoulder is an inherently unstable joint, the price paid for the mobility we enjoy. To successfully execute a strike, the shoulder must be stable and it must be attached to the torso to deliver a blow that resonates from the ground. All the good footwork and spine alignment are wasted if the shoulder is not stabilized. Without this stabilization all the energy that you are attempting to deliver into the body of your attacker is lost as the shoulder moves backward upon impact.

Shoulder drop from front   *Shoulder dropped from rear*

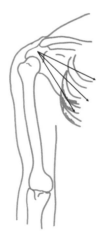
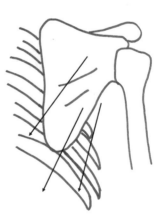

Even the slightest movement of the shoulder will waste this energy. It is important also to note that bent elbows or wrists also serve as places for energy to escape from the strike as well.

Body drop

An aikido instructor I trained with was fond of the phrase, "Weight underside." At the time, however, I had little understanding of what he was talking about. My judo sensei stressed the importance of being on top of my opponent, and my karate sensei talked about getting heavy. Simply put, all three of these men were in their own way explaining that it was essential to martial arts that you control your own body weight and not allow your opponent to control his.

Once you have control of your own body you can then impose your will on your opponent in an explosive manner.

Sun Tzu had it right

In the book *The Art of War*, Sun Tzu states, "Thus we may know that there are five essentials for victory:

(1) He will win who knows when to fight and when not to fight.

(2) He will win who knows how to handle both superior and inferior forces.

(3) He will win whose army is animated by the same spirit throughout all its ranks.

(4) He will win who, prepared himself, waits to take the enemy unprepared.

(5) He will win who has military capacity and is not interfered with by the sovereign."

Sun Tzu's well-known saying is most applicable here: "If you know the enemy and know yourself, you need not fear the result of a hundred battles.'

To aid in aligning your body to control your weight you need to control your spine. To do this you must remove the spine's natural curve. It works like this: The design of the spine gives structure, yet flexibility, to the abdomen and the torso. Although it twists and bends throughout the day, your goal here is to lock it. A traditional karate spine set for combat does not absorb the bumps and nudges of the day; it becomes linked to the ground. This setting of the spine is best begun at the base of the spine in the lower abdomen at the Coccyx and Lumber #5, which were touched on briefly previously.

The belt drill This drill is used in our school to better understand the sensation when linking the torso to the abdomen. You will need two partners and an *obi,* a karate belt. The *obi* is wide enough to avoid injury and strong enough to take the stress you give it; a piece of rope or other material is not recommended.

• Take an obi and wrap it around your belly, back to front, which is likely the opposite way you learned to wrap your belt.

• Stand in a strong upright stance. If you are familiar with the stance *sanchin dachi*, then use it; if not, any strong upright stance you feel comfortable with will work.

• One person stands to your left and one to your right. They pull the ends of the belt so it cinches around your abdomen.

• Relax and let them pull a little more as you let the belt tighten around you.

• Take a deep breath into your back at the belt level. Do not fill your lungs and then push down into your belly, but rather breathe directly into your lower spine, straightening the lower lumbar region and expanding outward.

• Now, move your mind to the sides of your belly underneath the floating ribs and expand in this direction. Each instance of your concentration and expanding should cause your assistants who are holding the ends of your belt to be pulled further inward to your center.

• Finally, expand the front of your belly outward and link all four directions.

The sensation from this drill demonstrates the way your belly functions when fighting in traditional karate. This is the technique that links the lower body, keeps the weight underside and allows even old men to absorb full-on body shots. Most importantly, though, this expanding of the body and linking of the spine serves as a platform to generate significant power.

Important point: The secret of true power in traditional karate lies not in the fist but in the *hara danden* or, center point of the body. And such actions of aligning the spine, the entire skeleton, and then moving swiftly with no advance warning are highly effective acts that are small and unseen to the average person.

> The secret of judo lies in the little fingers
> and the little toes.
> - *Gunji Koizumi, paraphrased*

The makiwara

The makiwara is a traditional training device used in karate (see Chapter 6 for more details on how to use this device).

It is a simple post put into the ground or mounted to the floor with some sort of protective covering, leather, or a small pad, at striking height. It is a highly effective training tool, yet often misunderstood and misused.

The makiwara is not an instrument to toughen the body for fighting via the enlargement or scarring of the knuckles on the hand; rather, it is a tool to aid in the alignment of the body.

When you can efficiently transfer energy from the ground into a makiwara, you strike harder. The heel and the spine, as discussed, are two critical points of energy transference. These move from the first point (the ground and the heel), to the midpoint (the spine), and to the final contact point (the fist).

When striking the makiwara, it is important to transfer energy from the ground to the board. The single greatest indicator of good, solid transference of energy in a strike is the lack of a rebound when striking the makiwara. Here is how to audit yourself to see if you are transferring energy well, or not.

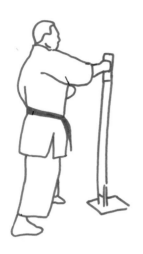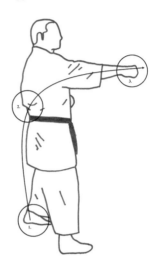

Hit the Makiwara several times and notice the rebound you are allowing, or even using, to re-chamber your fist as it comes off the board. Often a person will hit the board, extending it to a taut and bent position, then relaxes and allows the board to push his fist back for him to re-chamber for the next strike. This relaxing and rebounding happens almost instantly, preventing the full transference of energy into the opponent, or in this instance, the makiwara.

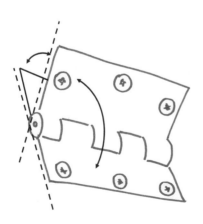

Using the imagery of a door hinge you can see that a locked-out door hinge can support a lot of weight. However, even the slightest shift from one side to the other will cause it to collapse under the weight. When striking the Makiwara your body should be like the door hinge, locked for the moment of contact and then relaxed. Strike the makiwara and hold the body-lock in position. This transfers the energy from your body into the target.

Keep the pressure on

Karate is designed to gain dominance and to keep pressure on the opponent until the altercation is over. Karate also does not allow for separation once contact is made. There is no hitting the other person in the face and waiting for a response like in the movies. One strike is followed by another form of attack – a push, a strike or other combination that is designed to keep the opponent off balance both mentally and physically until the fight is over. My judo instructor, Kenji Yamada, a two-time national judo champion back in the fifties, would say in a firm voice from across the dojo mat, "You gotta attack."

You can't just attack, however. You must study the means of attack and learn from the masters who have left their knowledge in the form of kata. Those who practice kata and study it will discover a wealth of useful information beneath the surface. They will see that blocks are not blocks but aggressive offensive moves, strikes always occur in multiples and at varying angles, space gets closed quickly, and dominance of the aggressor is achieved via a swift and powerful action or actions.

Traditional karate is designed to use everything at its disposal to end a fight, and an aggressive overwhelming force is the key component. Every criminal and every punk, unless he is under the influence of drugs, uses overwhelming force.

Hollywood got it right in the movie *Crocodile Dundee* when the main character, threatened by a mugger with a smallish knife, pulls out his huge bowie knife and announces the famous line, "You call that a knife? *This* is a knife."

Important point: Bigger weapons *are* better, and when it comes to hand-to-hand combat, better technique is the equivalent of a bigger weapon.

Giving a hit and taking a hit

Again, the key to understanding the true power of karate and all martial arts is to understand their deeper aspects, that is, the architecture of the body. If your body can take a direct blow and be undamaged, the architecture is correct. Taking a blow is a means of testing the very same architecture that is used as a platform to generate powerful body rattling strikes. An example of this ability is seen in Robert W. Smith's book *Martial Musings* where as a young man Smith is shown in a photograph striking Xingyi master Wang Shujin in the abdomen with no results.

History shows us that there has been and will always be violence in any society. Violence always happens faster than you think and harder than you assumed, with some level of surprise. The aforementioned precepts are no different today than they were 200 years ago. Nor are the key precepts of karate. Letting the lessons of history speak to us provides us with powerful tools for the inevitable violence that unfortunately "doesn't go away."

Kris **Wilder** began his martial arts training in 1976 in the art of Tae Kwon Do and over the years has earned black belt-level ranks in three arts: Tae Kwon Do (2nd Degree), Kodokan Judo (1st Degree) and Goju-Ryu Karate (4th Degree), which he teaches at the West Seattle Karate Academy. He has trained under Kenji Yamada, who as a judoka won back-to-back United States grand championships ('54-'55); Shihan John Roseberry, founder of Shorei-Shobukan Karate and a direct student of Seikishi Toguchi; and Hiroo Ito, a student of Shihan Kori Hisataka (Kudaka in the Okinawan dialect), the founder of Shorinji-Ryu Kenkokan Karate.

Though now retired from judo competition, Kris competed on the national and international level. He has traveled to Japan and Okinawa to train in karate and has authored several books on the martial arts, including co-authoring The Way of Kata. He has also written guest chapters for other martial arts authors and has had articles published in *Traditional Karate*, a magazine out of the U.K. with international readership.

Kris hosts the annual Martial University, a seminar composed of multidisciplinary martial artists. He also regularly instructs at seminars.

Kris lives in Seattle, Washington with his son Jackson. He can be reached via e-mail at: kwilder@quidnunc.net, or by going to: www.WestSeattleKarate.com.

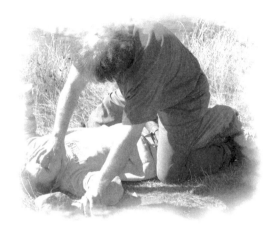

SECTION THREE

PUNCHES, KICKS, CLAWS, ELBOWS,KNEES AND A LITTLE GRAPPLING

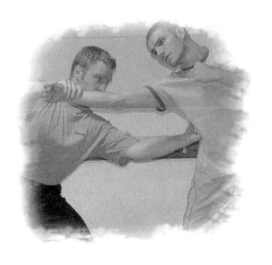

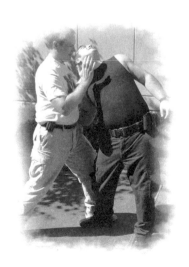

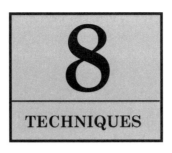

TECHNIQUES

9 Ways to Attack the Eyes: Intimate Brutality

By Loren W. Christensen

While this chapter is about attacking the eyes in a self-defense situation, let's begin by talking about the psychological side of killing. The similarity will be apparent in a moment.

Let me begin with an excerpt from the Pulitzer prize nominated book *On Killing* written by my friend and sometimes coauthor Lt. Col. Dave Grossman. Col. Grossman writes extensively in *On Killing* and in *On Combat,* the book we coauthored together, that within every *healthy* human being there is a resistance to kill another human being. Many studies have shown this to be true but it's beyond the scope of this chapter and indeed this book to examine them all. I will say that part of the evolution of weaponry – progressing from cavemen beating each other with bones, to spears, bows and arrows, armies, chariots, gunpowder, ships, jets, missiles and bombs that can crush the planet – has not only improved man's mechanical ability to fill military graveyards, it has also vastly improved his ability to overcome his psychological resistance to doing it. It's relatively easy to kill at a distance – missile range, artillery range, and rifle range - but it's a whole other thing to kill with your bare hands when you're standing nose to nose with an attacker.

Although it's a lesser act, there is also a tremendous resistance to attacking another person's eyes. We will talk more about this in a moment, but here is what Lt. Col. Dave Grossman writes about it in *On Killing*.

"Hand-to-hand combat"

an excerpt from
On Killing: The psychological cost of learning to kill in war and society

By Lt. Col. Dave Grossman

At hand-to-hand-combat range the instinctive resistance to killing becomes strongest. While some who have studied the subject claim that man is the only higher-order species who does not have an instinctive resistance to killing his own species, it's existence is recognized by almost any high-level karate practitioner.

An obvious method of killing an opponent involves a crushing blow to the throat. In movie combat we often see one individual grab another by the throat and attempt to choke him. And Hollywood heroes give the enemy a good old punch to the jaw. In both instances, a blow to the throat (with the hand held in various prescribed shapes) would be a vastly superior form of disabling or killing the foe, yet it is not a natural act; it is a repellent one.

The single most effective and mechanically easiest way to inflict significant damage on a human being with one's hand is to punch a thumb through his eye and on into the brain, subsequently stirring the intruding digit around inside the skull, cocking it off toward the side, and forcefully pulling the eye and other matter out with the thumb.

One karate instructor trains high-level students in this killing technique by having them practice punching their thumbs into oranges held or taped over the eye socket of an opponent. This procedure of precisely rehearsing and mimicking a killing action is an excellent way to of ensuring that the individual is capable of performing the act in combat.

In the case of the orange held over the victim's eye, the process is made even more realistic by having the victim scream, twitch, and jerk as the killer punches his thumb to the hilt into the orange and then rips it back out. Few individuals can walk away from their first such rehearsal without being badly shaken and disturbed by the action they have just mimicked. The fact that they are overcoming some form of natural resistance is obvious.

Tracy Arnold, an actress in the X-rated (for violence) movie *Henry: Portrait of a Serial Killer,* passed out twice during the filming of a scene in which her character was portrayed stabbing a man in the eye with a rat-tailed comb. This is a professional actress. She can portray killing, lying, and sex on the screen with relative ease, but even the pretense of stabbing someone in the eye seems to have touched a resistance so powerful and deep-seated that her body and emotions – the tools of the professional actress – literally refused to cooperate. In fact, I cannot find any reference to anyone in the history of human combat having ever used this simple technique. Indeed, it is almost too painful to think of it.

I believe that for a lot of people, even seasoned martial artists, the act of attacking another's eyes is viewed, as I've often heard people say, as "abhorrent," "detestable," "wrong," "icky," and "not fair." It's true! Some have said it's "not fair!" I've especially heard these comments coming from females during self-defense seminars where we have examined typical scenarios of women being attacked in parking lots, at ATM machines, and at their apartment doors.

Now, these women didn't have any problems slamming a hard foot between a mock assailant's legs in class (in fact, most did it with zest and a scary little smile on their faces) and pounding the bottoms of their fists onto attackers' noses (both targets represented by striking pads). But when it came to pretending to poke their fingers into the eyes of another student playing a bad guy, they balked. It was as if their hands, shaped like tiger claws, suddenly froze in the air two feet away from the baby blue target.

I've found most male students to be a little more aggressive, but not by much. Actually, I think they might just be better at camouflaging their distaste for the technique. While they flick their fingers at their training partners' eyes, they do it with considerably less mental and physical intent than when driving home a roundhouse kick to the stomach.

The exceptions

I have found that those female students with a history of physical victimization have fewer qualms about training to attack the eyes. Of those, the most ferocious have been victims of sexual abuse. Indeed, they claw and rip the target with a determination that says, "This time I'm going to win."

It can be hard to target the eyes. For sure, there is something intimate about touching that wetness that is a window to the soul and a pathway to the innards of the skull. We all know the agony of getting something in our eyes, the discomfort of when they hurt from fatigue, from allergy, and from a headache. To most of us, there is no horror greater imagined than to lose our sight. Perhaps it's a horror easily projected onto others, even those who would do us harm.

Mental conditioning

But it's such a great target, one that even the biggest assailant succumbs to. "Ay, there's the rub," to quote Shakespeare. The unarguable fact is that to strike the eyes is painful and demoralizing to an assailant. The rub, or the obstacle, is what we must do to overcome our resistance to striking this excellent target. One answer: *think fruit.*

Oranges Short of finding a village peasant to volunteer to let you gouge out his eyes for practice, you need an alternative, something that comes close to the real thing and helps to condition and enable you to strike the eyes without queasy qualms. You need fruit, juicy fruit with pulp. Lt. Col. Grossman mentioned oranges in the above excerpt from *On Killing*.

In my DVD, *Vital Targets: A Street-Savvy Guide to Targeting the Eyes, Ears, Nose, and Throat,* I demonstrate how to use oranges to simulate the feeling of sticking your fingers into the goo of another's eyes. My training partner slips on a pair of goggles to protect his eyes from the stinging juice and lies down on his back. He places two peeled oranges over his eye sockets and waits for my thumb attack from behind. I kneel on the floor behind his head and then, without fanfare, gouge my thumbs into the oranges. As my partner screams and writhes in pretend agony, I stir my thumbs in the juicy pulp and then rip them out the sides with admitted dramatic flair, complete with flying juice that covers my partner, the floor, and me.

Melons   Cantaloupe, watermelon, and honey dew are great, too.

- Slice a ripe melon in half, leaving in the seeds and pulp, and take it outside.

- Wear an old t-shirt or a raincoat. Any neighbors peeking through your shades are going to think you've lost your mind, so you may as well dress the part and put on a long raincoat. A hood isn't a bad idea either.

- Place the melon against a tree or against the side of your house, and hold it there with one hand. Form your hand into a claw.

- Plunge four fingers into the melon. Twist, gouge, and rip your hand out.

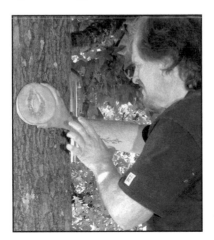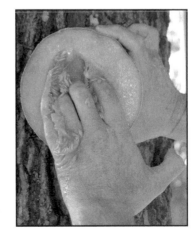

Isn't this a bit psycho?

Well, admittedly it is over the top, but it's fun and it provides you with some sense of what it feels like to completely gouge out a person's eyes.

Would you ever have to go to that extreme in a self-defense situation, to gouge, twist and rip? It would be rare, but not in a dire, life-and-death situation. Nor would it be rare for a soldier in desperate hand-to-hand battle with our country's enemy.

It's the mental conditioning, the desensitizing, that you want to gain from these fruity exercises. The sight of your partner kicking and writhing, the sound of his screams, and the feel of the wet pulp are all helpful in enabling you to scrape your fingers across the eyes and face of an assailant wanting to do you harm. You might never have to thrust your fingers into a person's eyes as deeply as you do the fruit, but by conditioning yourself to do so, at least to a limited degree, you will remove any hesitancy to quick-flick your fingertips against the eyes of someone deserving. The argument is that if you're desensitized to gouge deeply, you can scrape or poke superficially.

Attacking the eyes from behind

Lt. Col. Grossman writes elsewhere in *On Killing* that it's easier to kill an adversary with a knife from behind than it is from the front where you can see his face. Grossman writes:

> "The eyes are the window of the soul, and if one does not have to look into the eyes when killing, it is much easier to deny the humanity of the victim...The victim remains faceless, and one never needs to know one's victim as a person. And the price most killers have to pay for a close-range kill – face terrible, twisted in pain... this price need never be paid if we can simply avoid looking at our victim's face."

For some, there are two issues of concern: the feel of another person's eyes on one's fingertips and the look on the recipient's face, before, during and after the technique. Research, anecdotal evidence, and even common sense tell us that it's easier to attack an enemy from behind where you don't witness their "face terrible, twisted in pain."

When the attacker is standing   So does that mean you should make an effort to strike an attacker's eyes from behind? In my not so humble opinion, I say no, unless the opportunity is handed to you on the proverbial silver platter. An attack, in most cases, is sudden and unexpected, two variables that don't provide a lot of time for you to think, *I'll scamper behind this guy, reach over his head, and do a three Stooges eye poke on him.*

Unless you train otherwise, you are most likely going to react to what is directly in front of you. He attacks; you counter. During the course of the battle you might inadvertently get behind him, in which case you want to take advantage of the moment and attack his eyes. Of course, that thought or reflex isn't going to be there unless you have trained for it. However, if you specialize in getting behind your opponent as often as you can, the opportunities for you to strike the eyes from behind are going to be greater.

My personal style is to get behind my opponent as quickly as I can.

- Then I attack the back of his legs, his kidneys, spine, brain stem, and his eyes.

    o   Sometimes I hit all these targets; sometimes one or two: sometimes just the eyes.

- If the attacker is my height or shorter, I pull him toward me, reach over his head and make like a windshield wiper on his eyes.

- If he taller, I reach around the side of his head and rake his eyes.

- If he begins to turn his head right in the middle of my technique, I claw his eyes anyway, but with less reach involved.

When the attacker is on his belly   The same psychology occurs when the attacker is on his belly. You can't see his face, his eyes, or his agony. Attack his eyes, scramble to your feet, and flee while he writhes in pain.

Medical implications

Technique: Gouge: A thumb, or one or more fingers thrust into the eyes

- Implication: Depending on the severity of impact, the effect can range from:

  o   discomfort

  o   pain

  o   hemorrhaging: superficially or into the eye

  o   lacerations to the iris

  o   lens and retina can be displaced

  o   displace entire globe

  o   severe damage to the orbital floor

Technique: Rake: Thumb, or one or more fingers drag across the eyes

- Implication: Depending on the severity of the rake, the effect can range from:

  o   discomfort

  o   pain

  o   scratched cornea

  o   injured iris and pupil

  o   snagged cornea, iris or lens

- Blinded: If the eye technique is especially powerful or other conditions exist, it's possible to blind the recipient. It's even possible to pull the entire eye globe out of its socket. "Once the eye is dangling on your cheek," one medical technician said, "chances are it won't be seeing again."

You got to sell it to the jury

You're on the stand in court trying to convince a jury of retired school teachers and librarians how ramming your thick, hairy fingers into your assailant's eyes was the right thing to do. This isn't an easy task because many jury members share that same psychological abhorrence to attacking the eyes as we have been discussing. Even in a self-defense situation.

Be justified to impact an assailant's eyes and then, should you have to go to court, talk it over with your attorney as to how best to express yourself regarding the choice you made.

Techniques

If only all techniques in the martial arts were as easy to do as are those that target the eyes. After all, an insect that flies into your eye can make you yelp in pain, and a baby's finger that finds its way into your eye can give you several minutes of agony. So how hard can it be to counter strike an attacker's eyes? Well, it's a tad tougher than these two examples but not by much. All you need is an opportunity and a pathway to the eye(s).

Pathways

Hitting any target is about taking an unobstructed path from where your weapon originates to where the target is. In this case the weapon is your hand and the target is the assailant's eyes. If your hand is in the on-guard position next to your jaw and the target is three feet away just above the assailant's snarling mouth, the pathway is almost a straight horizontal line. All you need is the opportunity to send your hand on the path.

This is, of course, true of any technique you want to use – roundhouse kick to the chest or reverse punch to the face - but when thinking about attacking the eyes, you don't need to explode into the target with precise body mechanics, great momentum, and devastating power as you do with that kick or punch. With an eye technique, you only need a path to the eyes and a brief opportunity to hit not much harder than that flying insect or that baby's innocent poke.

Opportunity

This is a moment in time, sometimes only a half second in duration, other times longer, in which there exist a pathway to the target. Maybe your assailant dropped his guard when he attacked, maybe you knocked his attack aside, or maybe he glanced to the side for a moment to look at his buddy. These are opportunities.

Missed opportunities, like not dating that hot sophomore when you had the chance or not buying stock in Starbucks when it first started out are unfortunate. But not seizing the opportunity to fire an attack on an open pathway in a self-defense situation just might be your last miss.

Simple concept

Some readers will look at the pathway/opportunity concept and go, "Well, duh!" All fighting is about taking advantage of openings." I have two responses to this. First, if it's such a "well duh" moment, then why do so many fighters miss opportunities? Secondly, the concept is different with eye attacks because the pathway can be much smaller and the opportunity, time wise, can be much shorter than what is required with kicks and punches.

9 paths to the face

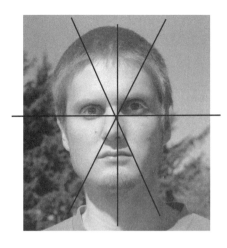 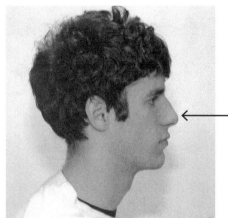

The lines that cross the face on the left represent angles of attack, or paths, to the eyes. Each line represents two directions. With the horizontal one, for example, you can attack the target from left to right or right to left. With the vertical line, you can attack the eyes from the high position downward and from the low position upward. The same is true with the two diagonal lines. Two directions on each of the four lines provide eight paths to the eyes. The ninth path appears on the face at the right: a simple straight path.

Let's look at nine scenarios in which you counter attack on one of the nine paths.

Straight in path   Your assailant reaches toward you with his left hand.

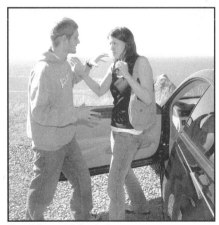 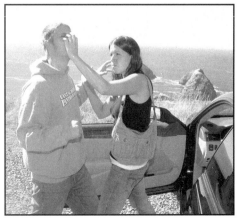

Backhand block it.   Quick jab his eyes with four fingers.

147

Straight down path   You're on top of the assailant on the ground trying to
control his right weapon's arm

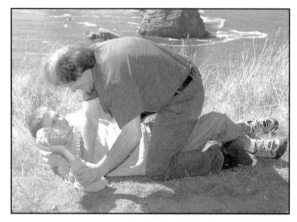

You struggle to control
his weapon's arm with
both your hands.

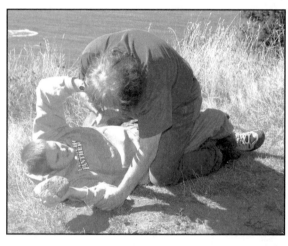

You snap your right arm up
to cover your head when he
starts to pummel it with his
free hand.

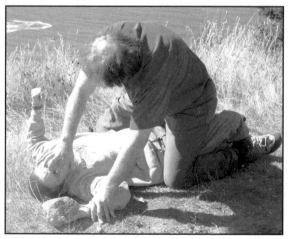

When he chambers to
punch again, drop your
claw straight down into his
eyes.

Straight up path You have knocked the assailant to his knees.

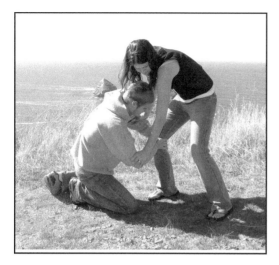

As you start to flee, he grabs your leg. You try to pry off his arm but you can't.

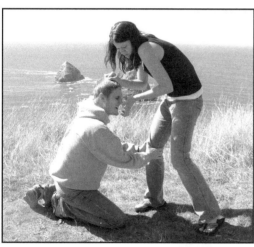

Grab his hair with your right hand.

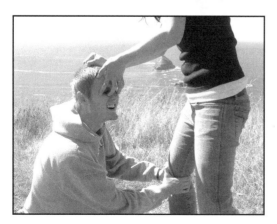

Rake your fingers straight up across his eyes.

Right to left path You're on your back on the ground and he drops down to finish you.

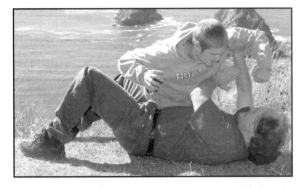

When he winds up a big left haymaker, palm-slam his upper arm.

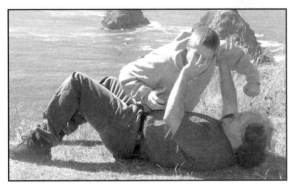

Rip your left claw across his eyes.

Left to right path He goes to smash you with a stone.

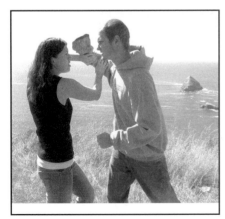

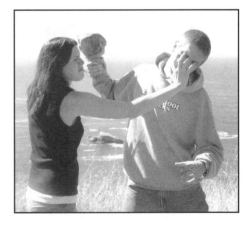

Jam his arm with both of yours.

Keep one hand there to control it and scrape the fingers of your other hand across his eyes.

Lower left to upper right path The assailant throws a sloppy right round kick at you.

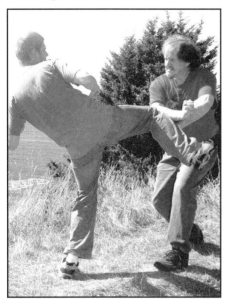

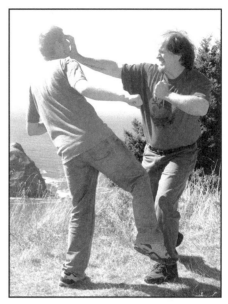

Block it.

Then lunge in with your closest hand to rake across the assailant's eyes.

Upper right to lower left path The assailant moves to slap you with his left hand.

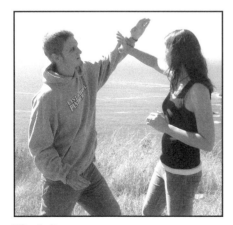

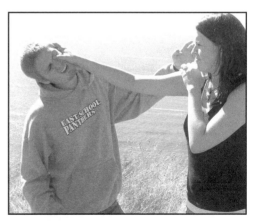

Block it.

Snap the same hand down the path and ram your right thumb into his closest eye.

Lower right to upper left path   The assailant throws a sudden left hook to your ribs.

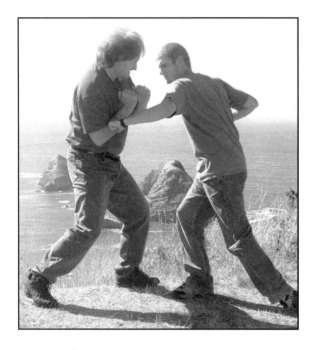

Quickly shield block with your arms.

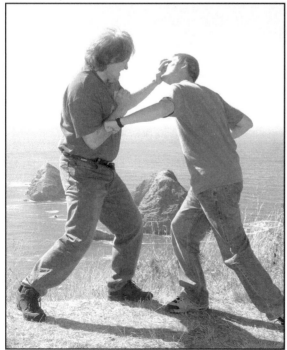

Shoot your left hand up and across your assailant's eyes.

Upper left to lower right path An assailant swings a can at you.

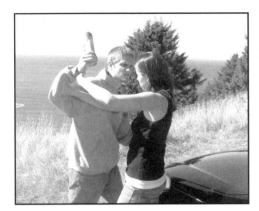

Block and grab his arm.

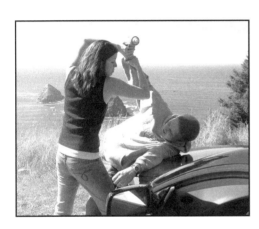

During the ensuing struggle, you muscle him over onto his back.

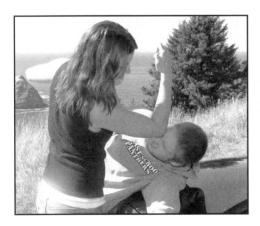

When the moment is right, ram the point of your elbow into his eye.

Shameless plug: In my book *Solo Training: The Martial Artist's Guide To Training Alone*, published by YMAA Publication Center, I list and explain several exercises you can do by yourself to improve the accuracy of your eye gouges and rakes.

Developing your ability to see the eyes as a target

If you train in a tournament style where punches and kicks are used to get points, or you're in a grappling style that emphasizes locking up the opponent, you will need to stress the eyes as a target in your training. If your teacher won't let you train to hit the eyes, consider getting together with one or two classmates to practice it.

Take any of your regular drills and add this caveat: you can only counter to the eyes. Yes, his knee might be open, or his groin, or his chest, but for now ignore them and become an eye hunter. Follow whatever path is open, sail past those other openings and attack the eyes.

It will only take a couple of workouts for you to see the eyes as an ever-present, target-rich place to hit. Then you can acknowledge those other openings, and hit them too, on your pathway to the eyes.

---

*L*oren W. Christensen's biography appears in the "About the Author" page at the back of the book.

Thanks to my daughter Amy Widmer and her husband Jace Widmer for demonstrating the techniques.

9 Ways to Target the Neck

By Loren W. Christensen

Most often, we think of our opponent's neck as a target to squeeze until its owner's face turns blood red and the eyes close in slumber (See Chapter 20 "Carotid constriction"). In this chapter, however, we're going to look at ways to impact the four sides of the neck to stop a dangerous assailant in a quick hurry. Because of the vulnerability of the neck and the potential for extreme injury, including death, you must be justified to target it. Sure, your brother-in-law's third beer has revealed his true, obnoxious side, but that is no reason to roundhouse your shinbone across his throat.

One more time: be justified.

Pathways

As was discussed in the last chapter on attacking the eyes, hitting the neck is all about taking advantage of an unobstructed pathway when it presents itself. When an opening appears, you must instantly move your weapon – hand, forearm, elbow, foot, shin or knee – and slam it into one side of your opponent's neck. That path might be a straight and horizontal one, upward or downward, or one of the four diagonal paths.

Opportunity

An opportunity is an instant, a hair of a second, five seconds if you're lucky, in which you can move on whatever path is available to hit the neck. If your attacker is an idiot, he might drop both his arms, stick out his chin, and taunt, "You want some of this, huh? Do yuh?" Or, you might be in a tight clinch with him when you sense a weakness in one of his arms. Or, as he blocks your escape route, he looks momentarily toward a noisy passing truck. These are opportunities and you must take advantage of them. *Now!*

Medical implications

There are volumes written on the implications of striking the neck. To keep things simple, know that a blow to the throat can damage the cricoid bone, windpipe, and an assortment of nerves. Blows to the sides and back of the neck can damage the spinal cord and vertebra. In extreme cases, such damage is simply called a broken neck.

On the low impact end of the spectrum, blows to the neck usually cause severe pain and a mild stunning sensation. At the severe end, a hard blow can cause structural damage, paralysis, and death.

Note: A light blow to one person might be a severe blow to another. This is why it's so critical that the situation justifies you impacting this vulnerable target. If the court deems the level of force used was not justifiable, you're likely to be imprisoned. However, if the situation did justify it, the technique just might save your life.

Decisions in life aren't always easy.

9 paths to the neck

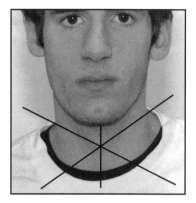

The four lines that cross the neck represent angles of attack, or paths. The beauty of the eight lines is that you can attack in either direction on any one line. For example, you can attack from lower left to upper right and you can attack from upper right to lower left. That gives you two directions per line for a total of 8 paths.

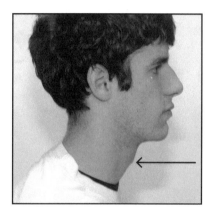

The 9th path is straight into the target (you don't get two directions on that one because you would have to start at the opponent's neck and then attacking yourself). While the photos depict face views, the 9 angles apply no matter which way the opponent is facing.

Besides attacking in either direction on a given cross line, you can attack with whatever weapon is available given your body position. For example:

A horizontal line (path) opens to the opponent's right side

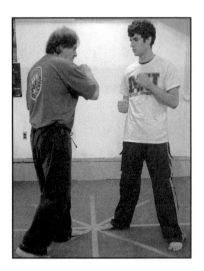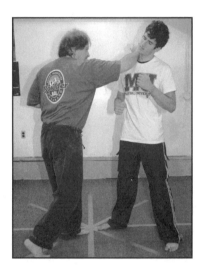

Because you're turned slightly to your left when the opening occurs, you can attack it with a right forearm strike.

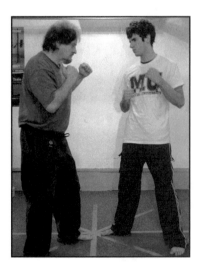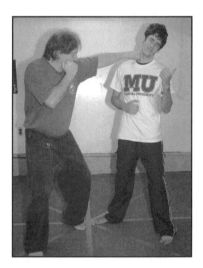

This time you're turned slightly to your right, so you attack it with a left hook punch.

A straight upward path opens to the front of the neck

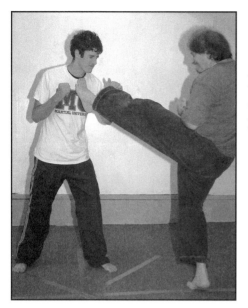

Because the opponent is bent forward slightly and within your kicking range, you hit his neck with a left front kick.

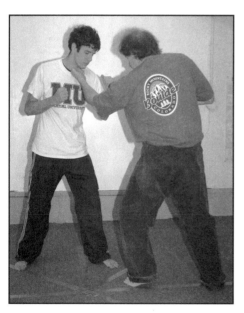

This time he is bent forward within your arm reach, so you drive in a right uppercut punch.

9 paths, 9 scenarios   Let's look at 9 scenarios in which you counter attack on one of the available paths.

Note: There are clearly other targets available in these scenarios, but since we're discussing the neck that is the only one you're going to hit right now. Limiting your targets helps to ingrain the concept of neck hitting into your mind. Once it has become an instant target for you, you can hit other open ones – groin, stomach, chest - on the way.

Straight in path

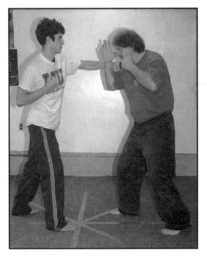

You execute a right backhand block against your assailant's left punch.

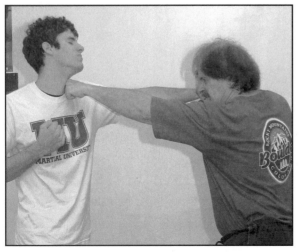

Follow with a left cross to his throat.

Straight up path

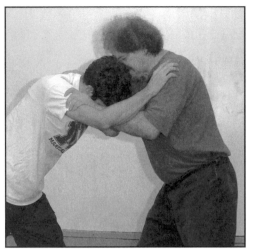 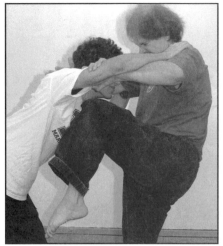

You're in a tight clinch.

Suddenly you're able to shift your balance and drive a knee up on a straight path to his throat.

Straight down path

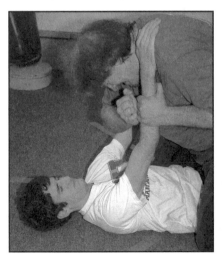 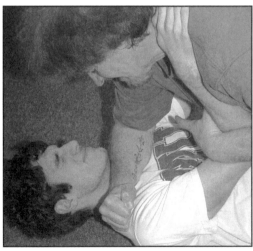

You're on top of the assailant on the ground and he is pulling you down onto him.

Don't resist but drop down and slam your forearm across his throat.

Right to left path

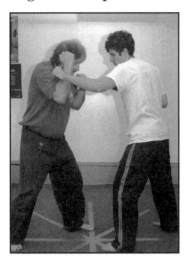 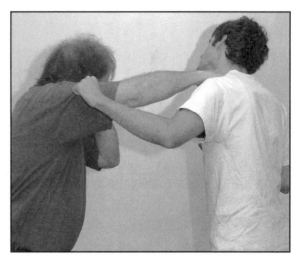

Right shield block his left hook to your head and then...

drive your right fist into the side of his neck.

Left to right path

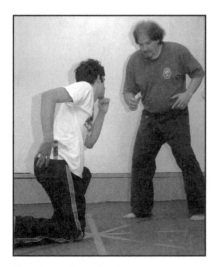 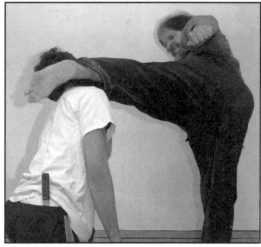

You have knocked your assailant down to his knees but before you can get past him, he reaches for a weapon.

Whip a fast roundhouse shin kick into the side of his neck.

Brachial plexus

There is a long complex explanation as to what all is involved with the brachial plexus and the interested reader is encouraged to research it. For our purpose, all we need to know is that it's a cluster of nerves on each side of the neck, roughly halfway between the side and the front. It's an amazingly reliable target area to affect a stun, even a knockout.

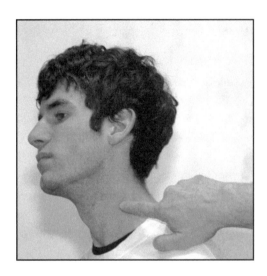

You can hit with just about any weapon: fist, either side of your hand, hammer fist, forearm, and even your thumb when used to poke hard. Now, some instructors say that the brachial plexus responds only to solid, penetrating impact, as opposed to a snapping impact, such as a snapping backfist. That has been my experience though one instructor told me that he had recently buckled his sparring partner's knees with a light, snapping blow to the target.

I suggest that should you want to use a snapping blow, allow the technique's energy to penetrate before snapping it back. This means the blow will stay on target a hair of a second longer than the typical tournament-style snapping blow.

To be able to write about it, I had a student strike my right brachial plexus with his forearm (yes, I am a hardcore reporter who sacrifices his health to bring you accurate information). On a scale of 1 to 10, 1 being the lightest blow,

I was struck with a 1, maybe a 2. I experienced these things:

- a blinding white light, like a flash from a camera.

- I fell back onto a sofa.

- I was told my eyes rolled back.

- incredible pain in my neck and shoulder.

- loss of motor activity, especially on the side struck and especially the arm.

- an inability to think clearly for a few seconds (but my thoughts were clear enough to know that I didn't want to do that again).

A harder impact will increase the intensity of these reactions and will likely cause unconsciousness. Be justified.

Note: I have heard of a few cases where the recipient didn't feel anything at all. One police officer said that in over 25 years of using the technique on the street, he came across only one person who tolerated it. It might be that a few people, for some reason, are invulnerable to it. Or perhaps the hitter simply missed the target.

Lower left to upper right path

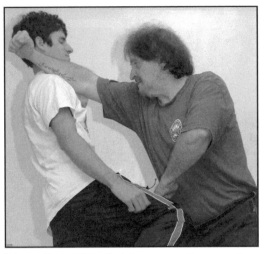

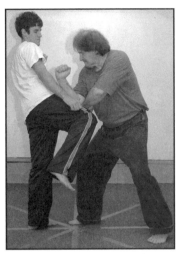

Then slam a hard right upper forearm into the side of his neck.

The assailant throws a right knee at you, which you block with both forearms.

Upper right to lower left path

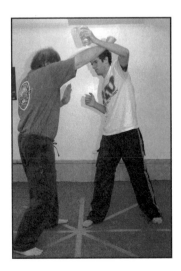

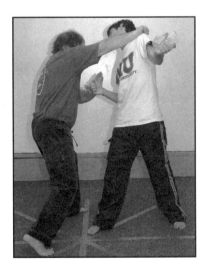

The assailant swings a drinking glass at you, which you block.

Drop step to the left and whip your right forearm down into the side of his neck.

Lower right to upper left path

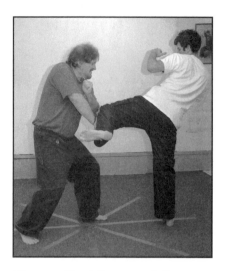

The assailant throws a left roundhouse kick at your ribs which you shield block.

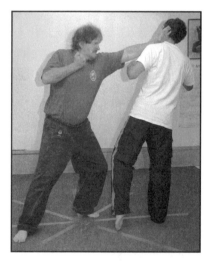

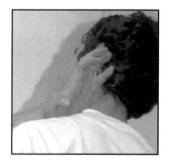

Strike with a chop into the assailant's neck cords.

Upper left to lower right path

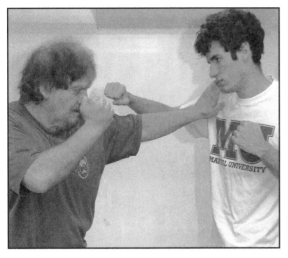

An assailant draws his right fist back, which you palm-check with your left.

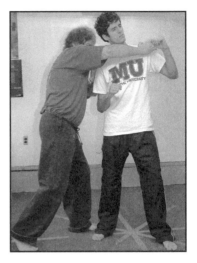

Pull his right shoulder and push his left to spin him.

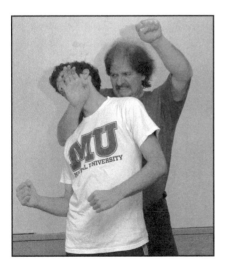

From behind him, use your right hand to pull his chin up to expose his neck. Stay away from his mouth.

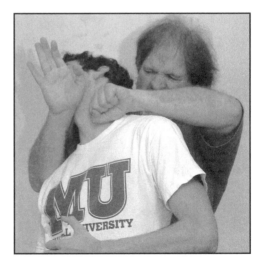

Slam your top fist repeatedly into his brachial plexus.

The shear

I picked this up from my friend Kris Wilder (see Chapter 7 "10 Ways to a Stronger Punch"), who likes to double the misery to the neck by employing a principle called "shearing." He creates this action by impacting both sides of the opponent's head simultaneously, but not straight across from each other. To shear, the impact points must be off-set a few inches. Here is how it looks.

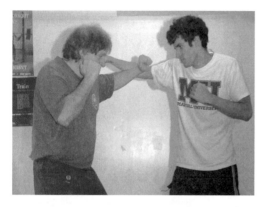

The attacker swings a wide, sloppy roundhouse at you.

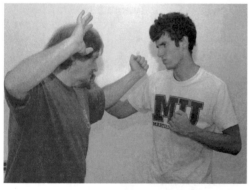

Block the attacking limb.

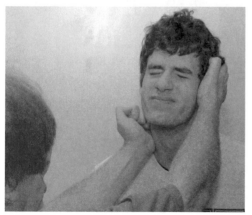

In one smooth, simultaneous action, slam your blocking fist into his brachial plexus as you simultaneously whip your other hand into a powerful slap against his ear. Because the ear is roughly three or four inches higher than the brachial plexus point, the off-set opposing impact creates a painful shear in the neck. This is in addition to the pain in his ear and in his brachial plexus.

Developing your ability to see a neck target

If you train in a tournament style where punches and kicks to the body are emphasized to get points, or you're in a grappling style in which the emphasis is on locking up the opponent, you will need to emphasize the neck as a target in your training so that you don't miss opportunities to hit it in a serious self-defense situation. If your teacher won't let you train to hit the neck, consider getting together with one or two classmates to practice.

Take any of your regular drills and add this caveat: you can only counter to the neck. Yes, his knee might be open, or his groin, or his chest, but for now ignore them and become a neck hunter. Follow whatever path is open, sail past those other openings and whack his neck. It will only take a couple of workouts for you to see the neck as an ever-present, target-rich place to hit.

Then you can acknowledge those other openings and hit them on your pathway to the neck.

---

*L*oren W. Christensen's biography appears in the "About the Author" page at the back of the book.

Thanks to Alex Larson for posing with me and to Lisa Christensen for her excellent photography.

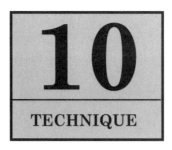

22 Ways to Defend Against a Dog Attack

by Loren W. Christensen

Note: Don't "test" these techniques on a dog or any animal to see if they work. It's cruel, it's illegal, and you could get hurt. The dogs were in no way hurt during the shoot. My veterinarian friend is a real person but to save his career he shall remain anonymous.

For 14 months of my three years in the United States Army, I served as a dog handler, patrolling with my German shepherd in the Florida Everglades. I got to tell you, that was more fun than a human should have. Every creepy crawly thing in existence lives in the Everglades, a horrible place where a young impressionable lad like me should not have been. It was so unpleasant that I volunteered to go to Vietnam just to get out of there.

Besides being on constant guard for deadly scorpions, alligators, and snakes, dog handlers in the Everglades worried about dog bites. While we ignored many of the Army's rules, we followed to the letter the many safety precautions set in place to prevent the immense pain of a German shepherd's bite.

Army dogs learn to be a one-handler dog, meaning that anyone else who ventures near is likely to have a German shepherd trot off with a bleeding chunk of his ripped out lung. We kept our distance from our buddies' dogs and felt quite safe with our own. We had each gone through eight grueling weeks of intensive training with our own shepherds in Texas and then worked 12-hour shifts with them at our duty station in the Everglades. Such an experience makes for a tight, loving relationship.

That's why I was so surprised when my dog took a serious bite out of my upper, inner thigh. (It even hurts to type *upper, inner thigh*.)

How much hurt is there in a dog bite?

A German shepherd's bite measures around 500 pounds of pressure per square inch, some dogs more, some less. Outside of the shepherd breed, the average dog's bite measures 150 to 200 pounds per square inch. Except for pit bulls.

Pit bulls trot with attitude because some of them can exert 2,000 pounds per square inch when they lock onto your privates.

Wolves can exert 1,500 pounds per square inch, should anyone ask.

We trained regularly with our dogs to keep their attack skills and their teeth deadly. One of the night exercises involved placing a human threat a few yards out into a field and then he would move from right to left to draw the dog's attention. Then when the dog's handler commanded, "Get 'em boy! Get 'em!" the dog went nuts: barking madly, straining at the end of his chain, his churning feet kicking up dirt and stones. In today's vernacular, the dog was in a "zone" where all he had on his mind was killing.

We learned from day one not to let the agitated and salivating dog circle behind us. Once he is directly behind the handler and then looks back toward the threat, all he sees are legs – the handler's. His somewhat domesticated, though still ancient brain, is in the zone and greatly agitated; the razor-sharp daggers he calls teeth are still craving bloody meat, just as did his ancestor's a hundred thousand generations ago. Then he sees legs. *Chomp legs*, his brain commands. *Me chomp legs now.*

That's how Fritz chopped into my inner, upper thigh – way too close to…I don't even want to think about it.

A half second after he bit, he realized his err. While he was sad and subservient, he wasn't as sad and subservient as I was. Nor was his pain meter blipping into the red zone as was mine. I didn't punish him because I was the one who messed up. He was just following his ancient dog ways.

Dog fighting "experts"

I'm going to go out on a limb here and say that there is no such thing as a card-carrying expert on how to fight a dog. Maybe you have fought a dog a couple of times but, in my not so humble opinion, that does not an expert make. If someone claims to have fought 50 dogs, they are either lying or their aftershave smells like a pork chop. Now, there are people who have had one or more experiences defending themselves against a dog attack, but that just makes them experienced, not expert. The reality is that we're all just white belts when it comes to fighting dogs.

My experience is limited to choking out several German shepherds and one Great Dane. As a dog handler, we learned how to pinch a dog's windpipe to get him to release his bite when the animal was so hyped, so in the zone, that it was no longer obeying verbal commands. Most often this occurred during attack-suit training when a frenzied dog wouldn't release from the sleeve and on rare occasions when one dog chomped into another because distracted handlers had moved too close to each other.

After I had gotten out of the Army, a buddy and I were walking his Great Dane on the beach, unleashed. He often brought the monstrous dog to class, and it always gave us a laugh when it picked up one of the dumbbells off the weight rack in his powerful jaws and trotted about the school as if he had a chew toy. On the beach, I was just telling my friend that I didn't think it was a good idea to have him unleashed when the dog suddenly bolted like an over-sized cheetah toward a small poodle walking alongside an elderly woman.

The Great Dane covered the distance in five seconds but it took us 20 seconds to get there, long enough for the giant dog to have a serious clamp over the poodle's entire mid body. As the woman screamed and the poodle gurgled, my friend froze in fear. I was just fresh out of the Army and dumb enough to straddle the Great Dane (not recommended), reach under its neck, and pinch its windpipe until he released the little dog. It was bad news for the poodle and could have been bad news for me should the Dane have bucked me off and went for a counter strike. The woman took off carrying her limp dog and we never saw her again.

So does this make me an expert at fighting dogs? No. It does mean I have experience at choking them out and that I've been real lucky not to have been bitten in the process.

Dog owners

While this chapter is about defending yourself against a dog attack, it's important to comment on some of the owners of these pets. The reasons people get a dog or several dogs, are varied: companionship, a live burglary alarm, personal protection, ego enhancement, and to get attention. Some are good owners and some are not. Sometimes a good owner, through ignorance and erroneous information, will inadvertently cause their dog to be mean. Sometimes a bad owner will make his dog turn mean through cruelty, inattention, or by virtue of the dog becoming reflective of a mean owner's personality. What does it mean for a dog to be reflective of his mean owner? Let me paint a picture. It's a cliché, but stay with me.

The stare

I've talked in other books about "the German Shepherd stare," a type of behavior sometimes exhibited by violent mentally deranged people and occasionally those whose rage has taken them to a dark place in their minds. It's a behavior similar to what an enraged dog does. As the person's body faces toward you, his head turns slightly to the side and his eyes transfix, wet, wide, and burning a hole through the floor. Every time I encountered such people when I was a cop, I never found that any of the psychology 101 tricks taught in the academy snapped them out of it. If you should ever run into someone like this, my advice is that unless you're a cop and you have to deal with the person, just back off slowly, and then run.

I call it the German shepherd stare because I saw it often while working with German shepherds. I would guess, however, that it's something that virtually all dogs do. When do they do it? About five, maybe ten seconds before they go for your jugular if they are big, your ankle if they are a small.

Psychology 101 for dogs doesn't work either. You can say, "Good dog," "What a pretty doggy," and "Whose my baby?" all day long and it won't likely snap him out of it. He just wants a treat: You.

The classic bad owner

It's the most rundown house on the block, complete with a weed infested, trash covered yard, a rusty truck on blocks, and a trashcan overflowing with beer cans. An unshaven 45-year-old man leans drunkenly on his broken porch railing, his filthy t-shirt stretched half way over his hairy beer gut, his work pants tattered and soiled with who-knows-what, and his bare feet long since washed.

As you walk past his house, he curses you in his smoke-graveled voice, though you don't know why. Then, from around the corner of his paint-chipped house, rockets a black, raggedy dog, part shepherd, part . . . wolf? Satan? His eyes seem like they have their own illumination, and it's blood red. His bark is more than a bark: it's mad, insane, and desperately hungry. A second before the dog finds the hole in the fence a few feet from where you stand petrified a thought passes across your brain: Sometimes a dog and its owner do look like each other.

Exaggeration? Not even a little. There are similar settings and situations in thousands of neighborhoods. Now, there won't be the scroungy-looking man in an upscale Beverly Hills-like neighborhood, but there is likely to be a tan, fashionably-dressed person, fit from his sessions with a personal trainer, accompanied by his lithe, muscular Doberman pincher. The man might be dapper, but his personality is similar to the scroungy man's. And so is his dog's.

Some owners take it personally

How serious are some pet owners? A few years ago in my community, several people lost their lives to pit bull attacks within just a few months. In response, a friend of mine wrote an expose for a local newspaper about the danger of pit bulls and their owners. Within two days, he and his newspaper were inundated with death threats. When angry pit bull owners began calling his home, he asked to stay with me for a few days until everything blew over.

It's indeed common for an aggressive dog to reflect its owner's personality. This is important to keep in mind should you want to confront an owner, say, in a park, because the dog is running about unleashed. Or, you want to go into the neighbor's yard to talk to him about his aggressive dog that runs loose in the street. You need to consider the situation, the nature of the dog, and consider what you know about its owner before you proceed. When your common sense tells you to refrain, do so. Then call the police.

Owners are liable

In the past several years, several states have passed laws with heavy penalties for the owners of dogs that hurt or kill people. In more than a dozen states, dog owners are liable for their dogs' behavior, while in the other states they are liable only if the owners knew or should have known that their dogs had a propensity to bite.

You might recall a landmark case that occurred in January of 2001, when two Presa Canario dogs (an especially large, ominous-looking dog that some believe were created in the 18th century for dog fighting) attacked and killed a woman in the doorway of her San Francisco apartment. The owner of the dogs, a San Francisco lawyer, was convicted of involuntary manslaughter and for keeping a mischievous dog that killed a person. She received four years in prison and became the first Californian convicted of murder for a dog's actions. Her husband was convicted of two lesser charges but was also sentenced to four years.

Important point: Over 80 percent of dog bites happen when the dog is with its owner or on its owner's property.

Scary statistics

According to the Centers for Disease Control and Prevention, there are approximately 4.7 million reported dog bites per year, which cost the property/casualty insurance industry roughly $317.2 million in 2005. Half of these injuries occurred on the dog owner's property.

Insurance companies can charge more for specific breeds of dogs that statistics show cause the most injuries and fatalities. According to a 20-year study of dog bite-related fatalities, here are the dogs most responsible, in descending order:

- Pit bull
- Rottweiler
- German shepherd
- Husky
- Malamute
- Doberman pinscher
- Chow Chow
- Great Dane
- Saint Bernard

Little dog bites hurt, too

While Rottweilers, Great Danes, German shepherds, huskies, pit bulls, bulldogs, boxers and Dobermans are all capable of removing large chunks of meat from your body, little lap dogs can do some serious damage to your ankles and calves. The problem is that you look like a real meanie when you fight a Chihuahua. But what are you going to do, sacrifice your ankles for the sake of political correctness?

One time I responded to a police call to a house where I had to walk up 12 steps onto a small, open porch. The door to the house was open, and when I knocked, a Chihuahua-type dog streaked out the door and ripped into my pant leg with all the fervor of a starving Great White, a really small one. It happened so quickly that I didn't have time to think, though I could feel its chomping mouth closing in on my shin. First, my uniform pants and in three seconds its rat-like teeth would be feasting on my leg.

I made a simple flick of my toe without even lifting my foot, launching the dog off the edge of the porch. The little shark dropped six feet to the ground, landing on its side in a cloud of dust and a little yelp. Just then, its owner came to the door.

"Oh my -" the elderly woman cried, rushing down the steps. "What happened to my little darling?"

Not wanting to be bogged down in extra paperwork, I said, "Don't know, ma'am. It was the strangest thing. Your dog just ran out the door and right off the edge of the porch."

"But he's ran out onto the porch a thousand times," she said, lifting the stunned *little darling* that had a moment earlier been two seconds from plundering the innards of my tender calf.

"Maybe his balance is getting a little off kilter." I said with all kinds of sympathy. "Maybe you shouldn't let him run out the door anymore."

"Thank you, officer. That's good advice. You're very kind."

"Thanks ma'am. I'm here to serve."

Types of bites

During my Army tour with dogs, I witnessed three types of dog bites. We had our own descriptive names for them: typewriter bite, shake-a-rabbit bite, and pressure bite.

Typewrite bite

There was a hardcore Marine Gunny Sergeant in our dog training school. He hated us, we hated him, and his dog hated him more. One day, his dog turned on him and chomped into his right hand, then his forearm, and upper arm. He chomped at the Gunny's face but the man snapped his head back so that the dog's teeth clamped only air. Then he bit the Gunny's other shoulder, then proceeded down to his upper arm, his forearm, and then his hand. Sort of like an old typewriter: a Royal. A not so loyal Royal.

The next day the Gunny was in the mess hall with both arms in casts. One of the privates was feeding him as if he were a baby. I heard that he had to retire form the Marine Corps.

I'm so glad that when my Army dog bit me way up there on the inner thigh that he didn't do a typewriter bite.

Shake-a-rabbit bite

The dog clomps into you and then shakes his head back and forth so fast it's nearly a blur. What makes this bad is that each time he forcefully jerks his head to the right, left, up and down he is ripping and shredding your flesh - and enjoying every second of it.

Pressure bite

Remember, some breeds can bite with a 2000-pound grip. Think of it as applying pressure with teeth filed ultra sharp from hours of gnawing on bones. Those teeth, backed by the dog's powerful jaw muscles, can punch through skin, fat, muscle, tendons and bones.

Combination biters

Sometimes a dog will chomp a pressure bite into its target and, just when the victim wonders what could be worse than this experience, the dog answers by changing to a shake-a-rabbit bite. Or a typewriter bite.

At that moment, the dog is large, in charge, and free to vary his technique.

Where and how they bite

According to hospital Emergency Rooms, dogs have their favorite places to bite:

- 45.3% to the arm/hand
- 25.8% to the leg/foot
- 22.8% to the head/neck
- For children 4 years and under, 64.9% of injuries were to the head/neck.
- For those 15 and older, 86.2% of injuries from dog attacks were to the extremities.

Types of dog-related injuries recorded in Emergency Rooms:

- 26.4% as "dog bite"
- 40.2% as "puncture"
- 24.7% as "laceration"
- 6.0% as "contusion/abrasion/hematoma"
- 1.5% as "cellulites/infection"
- 0.8% as "amputation/avulsion/crush"
- 0.4% as "fracture/dislocation"

The good news, sort of In most cases (read: not all cases), dog attacks involve a quick bite, maybe a chomp.

Safety techniques

Tips to keep you from having to defend yourself against a dog attack.

- Ask the owner if it's okay to pet him

- Stay outside of the maximum length of its leash.

- Do not approach it suddenly.

- Extend the *back* of your hand and let the dog sniff it. Then pet it.

- Be cautious around a mother dog and her puppies.

- Be cautious of a dog that is eating or sitting protectively near a child.

- Do not stare a strange or angry dog in the eyes. Nor should you look down as that might be interpreted as being submissive and the dog will think you're an easy mark. Try to assume a neutral stance and look at him without affecting a hard (or frightened) stare. You want the dog to lose interest in you and go away.

- Be especially cautious around a dog that has a history of abuse.

- Do not corner a dog.

- Do not poke at a dog's face. Even a mellow, well-behaved dog will snap at you.

- No not startle or touch a sleeping dog.

- Do not ignore his bark.

- If a dog startles you, don't run or scream. Stand still with your arms at your side. When you run, the dog thinks you are escaping prey.

- If you sense that a dog is dangerous, respect your instinct.

- Speak with a soft, soothing tone of voice.

- If you're a jogger, skateboarder, roller blader, or engage in any other activity where you're moving quickly, try to avoid being near a dog, even one that's on a leash.

- Do not smile. The dog might perceive baring your teeth as a threat to fight.

- Back away slowly, one slow step at a time.

- Breathe deeply and *try* to remain calm. A dog can sense your fear.

- If a dog knocks you down, stay down, curl into a fetal position, and remain motionless.

Important point 1 : There is no such thing as a dog that doesn't bite. No matter what the owner tells you, no matter how cute and cuddly the dog is, it will bite if it feels like it.

Important point 2: Respect what the dog wants! If it's barking and snarling, he is communicating his definite displeasure with you and what you're doing. Challenge him and he will likely follow-up on his warnings.

Fighting techniques

Let's begin slowly.

Verbal commands

I've recently discovered that with my annoying neighbors' dogs – the house owners to the north have three dogs and the ones to the south have one – that if I shout in a deep commanding voice over the fences, "NO!" they stop barking. They don't stop for long, but the act does say something about the value of a commanding voice with dogs.

As a cop, I found that a commanding voice used on a fast-approaching dog – worked the handful of times I tried it. Now, most trained dogs know the command "Stay!" but all dogs know the powerful utterance "No!" which was the command I used. Of course, some might choose to ignore the command, but I was fortunate enough to use it on aggressive dogs that yielded to it instantly. Don't scream the command with all the desperation you're feeling at the moment, but give the word a strong, loud and firm voice.

Since trained dogs might know hand signals, you might also hold up your open palm as you shout "no" or "stay." Don't flail your arm about, which the dog might perceive as threatening. Just raise your arm slowly and slightly push your open palm at the dog as you give your verbal command. You might have to give the command several times.

If he stops, try giving him the command "Down!" or "Down, boy!" With the verbal command, move your hand from the palm up, fingers pointing up position to a palm-down position as if you were pressing something down. You're hoping the pressing motion will make the dog lie down, which he might do if he has been trained and is one to obey you.

Important point: Know that not everyone agrees with using hand signals. Some people suggest that you not raise your hands prematurely as it might antagonize the dog more and you will lose the benefit of your verbal commands. However, if it's a neighbor's dog and you know he has been trained in verbal commands and hand signals, there is a chance it will work. Should the dog appear to become more agitated by your hand, lower it slowly along your side and continue with only verbal commands.

If the dog doesn't react to your "stay," "no," and "down," know that you're facing a potentially dangerous dog, one that is definitely unpredictable.

Look for these traits

Dominant-aggressive traits (serious threat)

1) The dog wags its tail but not its hind quarters, he watches you intently, he's rigid, and his hair is standing up.

2) The dog closes his mouth between each bark, while its ears point at you like their dual gun barrels above two piercing eyes.

Subordinate-aggressive traits (less threatening)

1) The dog's mouth is open, teeth bared, ears back, head and tail low, and he avoids eye contact.

2) He lunges and retreats without getting too close.

The dog attacks

Your commands don't work; you have no avenue of escape; the dog takes you by surprise. Now it's three feet away and closing.

A small dog

The good news is that a small dog can't leap up to your neck and chomp into your Adam's apple, but the bad news is that it can give your ankles and calves some shredded misery.

Kick it. A solid blow to its nose, ribs or groin will stop the majority of lap dogs from sinking their tiny, but nasty teeth into your flesh.

Big dogs

There is no one solution to fighting a big dog, just as there is no one method to defend against a human attacker. So let's look at a few ways that have been successful and ways suggested by experienced dog handlers.

Assume a fighting stance   This offers you greater stability than standing flat footed with legs parallel with each other. When I trained dogs in the Army,

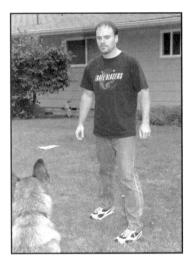

I saw 200-pound soldiers in thick, heavy attack suits get knocked flat on their backs when a shepherd leaped at them at full charge and slammed into their chests. Achieve stability quickly; you want to stay upright.

To protect your groin, consider turning your front foot inward slightly. Don't minimize the importance of this target (like you would, anyway) as it's a convenient one for dogs. If he circles you, turn with him and keep that lead leg ready to swing across your body to protect your groin.

Defensive stance   When an attack is imminent, cover your vital targets as well as you can.

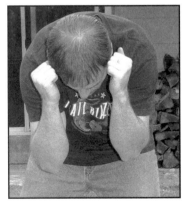

Maintain the staggered foot stance with your lead foot turned inward slightly to protect your groin. Hold your forearms vertically along your ribs to protect your sides and your abdomen. Position both fists along the sides of your head and be ready to protect your throat (when I was a dog handler in the Army, I trained my dog to leap at the neck).

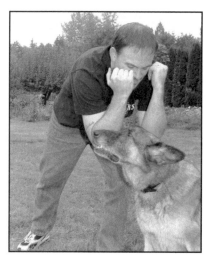

Rotate your upper body slightly, using your forearms to smack against the dog's charge, similar to how a cornered fighter uses his forearms to block and cover his upper body against his opponent's blows. Your forearms protect your vital targets while indirectly "offering" the dog your limbs. You don't want him to eat your forearm but most would say that is preferable to him eating your stomach or throat.

Rabies or, The fun just keeps getting better and better

Should you get bitten by a dog that is aimlessly running about attacking car bumpers, fire hydrants or any other stationery objects, and it has wild-looking eyes and a foaming mouth, he just might have rabies. If that news isn't bad enough, know that some rabies-infected dogs might not display these symptoms. Therefore, if bitten, visit your doctor immediately.

Rabies can be a fatal disease when left untreated. Try to get the dog quarantined – call the police, your local Animal Control office - so they can watch the animal for symptoms of rabies. If there is a possibility he is infected but he gets away, talk to your doctor about anti-rabies injections.

Some good news. Rabies shots used to be extraordinarily painful because the five-shot series was given through the abdomen. Today, you get them in the arm over a month's time. If your insurance doesn't pay, your injections will cost you around $1,500.

Defensive moves

The dog is charging toward you and you have three seconds to react.

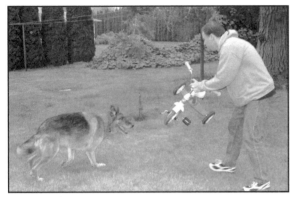

Feed him an object Should you be in the house grab a chair, skillet, lamp, or a potted plant. If you're outside push a trashcan in front of you, extend your briefcase, backpack, or a tricycle for the dog to bite.

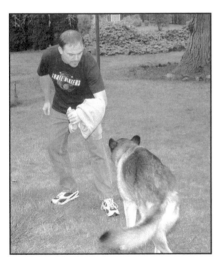

Feed him your padded arm If you're fortunate enough to have a few seconds, grab a blanket off the sofa, a bath towel off the rack, your coat off your back, or even your shirt, and wrap your left forearm if you're right handed, your right if you're left handed, and feed it to the dog. Will you feel the dog's bite pressure or his teeth through these things? Probably. I often felt the 200 pounds per-square-inch through the attack sleeve designed specifically to train dogs.

Feed him your bare arm   Never happen, you say? Well, that is a choice you will have to make: your arm or your stomach, your arm or your throat, your arm or your groin, your arm or your thigh. You might want to think about it right now because in the heat of the dog attack you might have only seconds to decide.

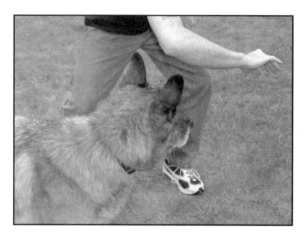

If you decide to do it, offer the dog the sides of the meaty part of your forearm. Muscle tears hurt, but there are a couple advantages over giving the dog your wrist bone.

When the dog has your relatively small wrist he will likely clamp down onto the bone reducing your chance to break free. It's also highly possible that the bite will damage the large blood vessels, nerves and tendons there. Worse case scenario is that you will bleed to death. A "better" case scenario is that you will

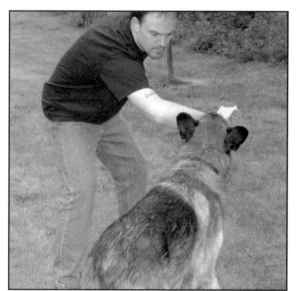

end up with nerve damage or have enough tendon damage that your fingers will no longer work.

Important point: When the dog has hold of the more fleshy part of your arm, there is a greater chance you can pull your arm out.

A dog's toenails

Keep in mind that toenails on a dog can do some damage - usually superficial, but blood running into your eyes or tearing one of your lips can be distracting.

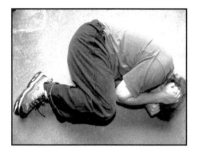

If you're on the ground, curl into a fetal position. Cover your head and neck. Lay perfectly still. Usually a still target is boring to the dog and they will retreat. Teach your child to do the same.

Offensive techniques

Many veteran dog handles suggest that you don't hit the dog, arguing that the more you fight it the more it thinks that you're prey. But you're the one under attack. If you deem it best to fight back, here are some things to consider.

Say the dog has hold of your shin. As hard as it is not to do, don't pull your leg away from the dog's clamped mouth. When you pull, jerk and twist your limb to escape the dog's horrific grip, you increase the damage the bite does to your tissue. Use all the intestinal fortitude you can muster and hold the limb still as you counter strike.

Is there a technique that works every time?

I posed this question to a veterinarian friend, who said. "Unfortunately, there are none," he said.

Forehead

While no one likes getting their foreheads struck, hitting a dog there won't do much, other than injure your hand should you punch it with your knuckles.

But if it's the only target available to you, and you have an especially powerful, well-trained palm-heel strike, hit the target multiple times.

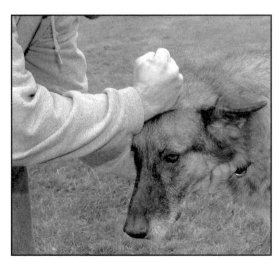

Better to pound the dog's forehead with a hammer fist. Here the dog's head is supported by the non-hitting hand. This is an option that creates a base so that the head receives the blow's full impact, but it's a risky one because the dog might bite it. But if at that exact moment during the scuffle your hand is in position, it's a consideration.

Nose

Smash your fist into its nose as hard as you can. Use your normal punching fist or your bottom fist, the hammer. Hit him as many times as you can, hard and fast. My veterinarian says that if the dog isn't a pit bull, smashing the nose works sometimes. *Sometimes.* "Dog's noses aren't nearly as sensitive as ours," he said.

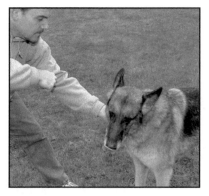

Here, quick-hands-Dan, my son, executes a fast punch to the dog's nose and a slightly circular punch below his ear. A combo is an option, but only if you have fast, strong hand techniques.

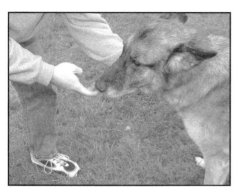

If you have strong fingers, consider clawing the nose. Try to catch its nostrils and rip it to the side. Don't stop with one claw; claw repetitiously, fast and furiously.

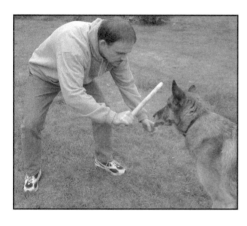

Sometimes – *sometimes* - whacking an aggressive dog's nose with a stick will make it back off.

Important point: A dog fears pain and the person who administers it to him. Most dogs, anyway.

Ears

Ear gouging   While sticking your fingers into a vicious dog's ears probably isn't your first choice of defense, if the pathway to it is open and it's all you have, do it. Ram one or two fingers in, form them into a hook, and rip them out. A dog hates that and he will likely jerk and twist in such a way that he will make available another target for you to hit or grab.

Twist or pull the dogs ears, and do it hard. As with ear gouging, at the very least you hope the twist will open a better target. At the most, you hope it makes him back off.

Punching or kicking the dog at the base of his ear at the side of its head is effective on some. A friend did that to a 100-pound Rottweiler and it knocked

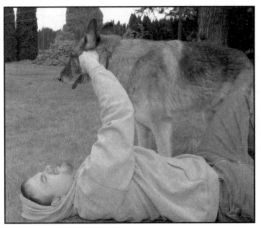

the dog down for a moment. My veterinarian friend concurs, saying that a blow there "... scrambles the inner ear a little. But it doesn't work on pit bulls. Actually, the dumber the breed is the less pain works and the more you need to disable them. Chokes, for example."

Eyes

I once read where a woman repeatedly poked a pit bull in the eyes but it was too busy chewing her poodle to notice. Of course, we don't know how accurately she poked the dog's eyes or with what force.

The veterinarian says, "With pit bulls, I doubt that eye gouging would help. Baseball bats and pipes to the head rarely do with them."

If the eyes are the only vulnerable target available to you, you can't be squeamish about it; you must attack them with extreme prejudice.

Don't think poke and don't think flick. Think *gouge*. Then think gouge *deeply*. The dog might be in a psyche zone that is so intense that he doesn't feel pain, but he still has to see. Then rip them out to the side.

Does ripping a dog's eyes sound severe? Yes. But can a dog's fangs rip and tear and disfigure and kill? Yes. Life is about choices.

Mouth

I know two people who have kicked at dogs' faces and both got their feet bit. You might have a fast kick, but have you seen how fast some dogs can move? The veterinarian says, "I don't recommend kicking to the face because dogs are expert at short, quick movements with their teeth. It's their best trick. All they do is adjust their angle of attack by a hair, and they have you."

You don't want to punch it either. A friend of mine did that and was rewarded with a handful of puncture wounds.

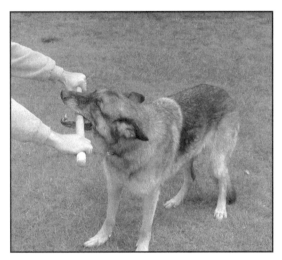

Some people have had luck with shoving a stick in a dog's mouth. Not vertically as cartoon characters do to alligators, but horizontally. Hold it at both ends and slam it in hard. Then twist it forcefully to the right or left. Depending on your strength, the dog's strength and size, and other factors, the hard twist might sprain the dog's jaw.

Chest

"There are two reasons to kick the chest," my veterinarian friend says. "One is to injure the dog or to get him to back off so you have time to regroup, run, or whatever."

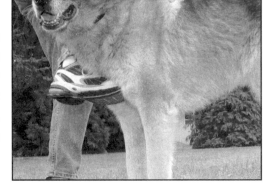

To injure the dog, kick right where the neck meets the chest. It's a vulnerable site in nearly every species because there is a lack of padding there. Besides pain, it can set off a cough reflex, thus distracting the dog.

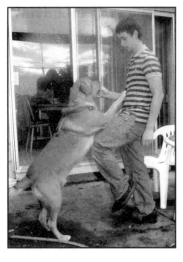

To knock the dog back and even knock him down, simply knee him in the sternum. The veterinarian says, "If you only need to get a dog off of you that is not super-intent on getting you, it is really easy, doesn't require lightning reflexes, and works almost every time. They usually land in a pile, too. The knee to the chest can really help people who have little skill."

Neck

Depending on the length of the dog's neck, this target can be easy to hit or difficult to hit. The brachial plexus point (the brachial stun technique on humans is discussed in Chapter 9 "9 ways to target the neck") on a dog is deep in the armpit, and thus hard to hit, unless somehow you are under the dog or he is standing on two legs and is totally vertical.

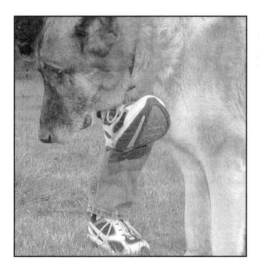

When you have an opening, punch or kick the dog hard in the throat.

Choking: Time to get up close and personal. Let's start with the windpipe choke, which is done by simply pinching it hard between your index finger and thumb.

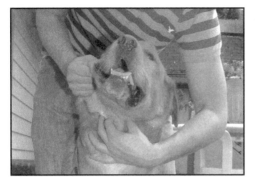

Avoid straddling the dog. I did it a few times and was lucky the dog didn't twist around and chomp me or thrash about so that I fell. That said, you might get away with it with a smaller dog.

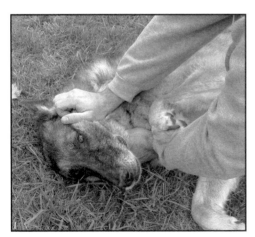

It's better to pinch the windpipe from the side of the dog. Grab handful of scruff close to the face. Be careful because some dogs can turn within their skin and bite you. Your other hand then slips under its jaw and pinches the trachea just below the dog's "voicebox." The cartilage around the voice box is too thick so you want to pinch just below it.

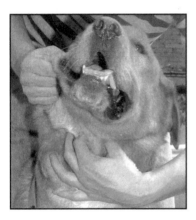

Dog lying on its side: Grab a healthy bunch of fur on the side of his face, or lean on the side of his face if he is a short-haired dog, and push his head into the ground as your other hand squeezes its trachea.

Jujitsu choke: This is somewhat unorthodox but when done right it's highly effective.

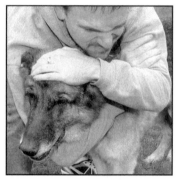

Don't do it this way. There is no pressure against the dog's windpipe when your elbow points out from under the dogs jaw.

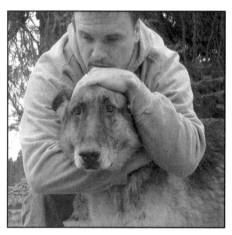

Do it this way. Your forearm extends across the dog's neck about midway between his jaw and his chest. Do it quickly from behind or from his side when he is somehow braced by your body, wall, tree, or anything that prevents him from twisting and chomping into your arm. Slip your forearm across the front of his throat, grab the biceps of your other arm, and use the hand of the arm to push the dog's head (and throat) forward as you pull your forearm back.

Important point: I asked the veterinarian what you should do after the choke has had its effect. He said, "I would suggest that if there is no avenue of escape and the dog is intent to kill, choke for at least 30 seconds past the cessation of struggling. If the dog does survive, it will be a bit of time before it has enough oxygen back in the brain to do anything." Take advantage of that time and get away.

Legs

Besides choking the dog unconscious, dragging a violent dog, face up or face down, by its back legs is considered by many experts as one of the best ways to get a dog from the attack site to a place where he can be secured in a room, outdoor shed, or some other kind of "lock-up." The trick is that you have to move fast from the moment you secure one or both back legs until you get the dog to where you're going to secure him. Move too slowly and the dog might thrash out of your grip or do a sit-up and bite you.

Grab the dog's rear legs, pull them up at least waist high, and back pedal as fast as you can to stretch them out. The more stretched, the less chance the dog will get you. (For some reason, neither of our big dog models would let us do this to them.)

Helping a victim of a dog attack

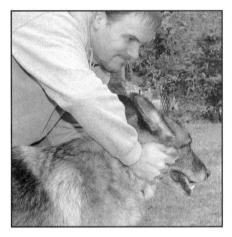

A violent dog begins stalking your child or another person in your presence. Here are some options when the dog has chomped down on someone and isn't releasing.

Option 1: Move quickly alongside the dog and grab his scruffs on both sides of his face.

- From here you can pull the dog away and/or...execute a windpipe choke as described above.

  o ....ram your fingers into its eyes. Repeat until it releases the victim.

  o ....force your arm into the dog's mouth. Your larger limb will force the dog to release the child's limb without tearing tendons and ligaments. This is painful, but if you can ram your arm inward and downward, you can minimize the damage the dog can do on your arm.

The dog attacks:

- Option 1: Run toward the dog screaming and yelling to distract it and force it to back away.

- Option 2: Do as described in Option 1 and when the dog releases the child, kick it hard in its side. Keep kicking until it backs away.

Two or more dogs

When there are two or more aggressive dogs, the one in front will try to distract you by moving in on you as the other dog, or several dogs, circle around and move in from behind. Clearly, two, three or six dogs are worse than one. You know you're having a bad day when a half dozen dogs rip into you and then simultaneously pull your body parts in six directions.

It's time to violate the passive suggestions mentioned earlier and get aggressive. Try to quickly identify the Alpha dog (the boss) and immediately charge after it. Your hope, and hope is about all that you have, is to frighten off the pack leader. If you can scare him off, the others will likely back down, too. Run at it yelling "No!" Keep advancing on him to hopefully diminish his fight. You must show aggression. Any weakness, any hesitation, will be sensed by the dog.

Keep in mind that dogs bite 4.7 million people every year, ranging from minor chomps to fatal maulings. Many adults and children, because of careless dog owners, have received horrific, permanent deformities from dog attacks. In a perfect world, dogs would be well-managed and people would not be injured and killed by them. But it isn't a perfect world and attacks happen.

Consider the ideas presented here, and research other techniques that have worked for people. Whenever you're around an unknown dog, heed the tips presented earlier as to what to watch out for. Be alert and be aware.

If you're a dog owner, be a responsible one.

---

*L*oren W. Christensen's biography appears in the "About the Author" page at the back of the book.

Many thanks to Dan Christensen and Brian Fitzgerald for posing with Zion and Buddy. The heroic photographer was me.

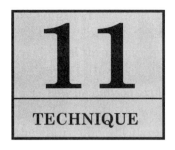

10 Ways to Execute Shock Blocks

By Lawrence Kane

"Try to understand this. If you wait for the attack, defend against it, and only then go in the attack by parrying and striking, you are making extra work for yourself. Moreover, there is always the possibility of missing the 'block.' If you approach the enemy with the attitude of defeating him without delay and with utter resolve then you will certainly be a better position to finish him off."

— Miyamoto Musashi

The reality of a real fight

Real violence sucks! If you lose a street fight, the result could be considerable pain, debilitating injury, disfigurement, or even premature death. If you successfully defend yourself, your attacker will often try to press criminal charges or pursue civil litigation, leading to significant expenses, adverse publicity and, oftentimes, irreparable harm to your reputation. You might spend time in jail or even in prison. There is also the potential of long-term psychological trauma should you maim or kill someone. Consequently, it is best to avoid fights. Unfortunately, you don't always have the option of walking away. Bad guys simply don't play fair. They cheat to win, attacking the weak and ambushing the unaware. Once they get the jump on you, bad things inevitably happen.

Working stadium security since 1985, I have witnessed or interceded in well over 300 violent altercations and I have yet to see a combatant try to throw only a single blow, even if he knocked out his opponent with the first strike (a rare occurrence). Assailants often move faster, strike more suddenly, and hit more powerfully than you would expect. Consequently, trying to successfully counter after an adversary has already ambushed you is extraordinarily challenging, particularly if you are already stunned, injured, trying to make sense of what just happened, or you are out of position from the force of his initial blow(s).

OODA Loop

Even if you manage to block the bad guy's first or second strike, there is inevitably another punch or kick already on its way. You are effectively behind the count before you even begin fighting back. To counter his offense, you need to (1) observe his motion, (2) orient, mentally digesting what is happening in order to formulate a response, (3) decide how to execute that response, and (4) act, performing a technique with which to defend yourself. It's a four-step process: observe, orient, decide, and act, or OODA Loop, as it's termed.

This process of observing, orienting, and deciding takes a certain amount of time, even a fraction of a second, before you can act in a coherent manner. As a flurry of blows comes in, it is easy to get stuck in the observe/orient stage, falling farther and farther behind as each new blow makes you begin the cycle over again. You see the punch, begin to formulate a response, get hit, and then see another punch or kick coming. Before you begin to respond to each new blow, you're already encountering a new situation. Consequently once you get behind in a fight it becomes progressively harder to regain momentum, particularly once you are injured or badly out of position.

Okay, that's the bad news.

Continuum of responses

The good news is that martial artists (*budoka*) can train to the point where they can near instantly react to a threat without much, if any, conscious thought. It's not easy to achieve that level of proficiency but over the long term all advanced practitioners eventually get there. In Japanese, this is often described as a continuum of responses going from *go no sen*, to *sen no sen*, and ultimately *sen-sen no sen*.

- **Go no sen** means "late initiative," blocking and riposting after an adversary has already attacked. Almost all new martial artists learn this method. It means to receive or block a blow and then to strike back. It is a great learning method, because it breaks advanced techniques down into small movements, but it is not practical on the street where you are likely to become overwhelmed by a determined aggressor. This is elementary martial arts (budo), abandoned quickly once any significant level of skill has been achieved. Unfortunately, if you miss an opponent's tell or you walk into an ambush, this is the best you can do at the beginning of a fight.

- **Sen no sen** means "simultaneous initiative," intercepting the adversary's blow just after it begins. This is an intermediate form of budo, using quickness and power to simultaneously attack and defend, cutting off the opponent's strike before it makes contact. This is where we begin to find street-worthy application. It is the minimum to strive for in a violent encounter.

- **Sen-sen no sen** means "preemptive initiative," cutting off a blow before it even starts. It looks an awful lot like a first strike yet is still a defensive movement. Practitioners sense that an attack will be forthcoming and then cut it short before the aggressor has the chance to transform his mental desire to attack into the physical movement necessary to execute that desire, in other words disrupting the bad guy's OODA cycle between decide and act. This is the ultimate goal of martial training insofar as self-defense is concerned; it is advanced budo.

Even better news is that a martial artist caught flat-footed or who has not yet developed the ability to respond preemptively with sen-sen no sen can still turn the tide and regain lost momentum in a fight. We can do that through blocks that act like strikes, movements that simultaneously protect us from harm *and* cause damage to our adversaries. I like to call them "shock blocks."

Be justified to hit first

Preemptive initiative (sen-sen no sen) can be problematic on the street. While it is very useful for keeping yourself safe, it also looks like you are the one who started the fight, particularly to untrained observers. Never forget that the majority of witnesses who may oversee your confrontation will have no experience with violence beyond the occasional movie or television show. It is prudent, therefore, to consider how your actions might look to an independent observer who might be called to testify about you in court.

Yelling something that sounds like you are a fearful victim rather than a crazed attacker may help. Consider shouting even as you strike. "Don't hit me," "I don't want to fight," "Get away from me," or "Help, he's attacking me."

As trained martial artists, we have an obligation to understand not only how to hurt someone, but also to know when it is appropriate to do so. If your adversary has the ability and opportunity to harm you, he places you in imminent jeopardy, and he leaves you with no safe alternatives other than fighting, you have a good case for the use of countervailing force in the eyes of the law. However, you must be able to articulate clearly how you knew your adversary was about to attack. You cannot just say that you had a feeling; you must be able to make clear to a police officer and a judge what tangible actions you saw that indicated he was about to attack.

Shock blocks defined

Before I describe how to execute shock blocks, it's important to point out that there really is no such thing as a block in traditional martial arts, at least not in the commonly understood sense. The Japanese word *uke* means "receive" rather than "block" as it is commonly, though incorrectly, translated. Your defensive technique receives the attack and makes it your own. Once you own the attack, you can do with it what you will. A fast, hard block, therefore, has the potential to drop an opponent in his tracks, ending the fight before you even need to throw what is commonly thought of as an offensive blow. The most successful of these applications keep you from getting hit while simultaneously stopping your adversary from continuing his attack.

A shock block in action

As you can see, focused, hard-hitting blocks are really attacking techniques, causing pain and disruption to the assailant so that you can retake momentum. I saw a great example of this type of defense during an altercation at a college football game. A drunken fan of the visiting school (whose team was losing) became belligerent, jumping up and down on the bleachers, taunting a home team's fan who was standing one row behind and slightly above him, and screaming obscenities at the crowd.

I had noticed the escalating confrontation, but before I could gather a team together to react, the drunk spun around and threw a roundhouse punch at the other man, putting all his weight into the blow. In one smooth movement, the other guy shifted slightly and executed what looked like, from my vantage point some 50 feet away, just a basic block.

 The result, however, was far removed from any basic technique. The drunk staggered forward, let out an ear-piercing shriek that I could easily hear over the roar of the crowd of 72,000, and collapsed to his knees clutching his injured limb. The man who executed the block saw us coming, rushed down the stairs, held his arms placatingly in front of himself, shouting something along the lines of, "Hey man, I never punched him," and beat a hasty retreat out of the stadium, no doubt thinking that we were about to arrest him. I actually did not intend to do that, but he bailed nevertheless. His erstwhile attacker turned victim, on the other hand, was not so lucky. He was rushed to the emergency room to deal with his dislocated elbow and subsequently arrested (beyond the physical altercation he initiated, he was also underage and quite drunk with a blood alcohol level well over twice the legal limit).

When receiving attacks from an adversary, most classical martial systems use a check/control type of methodology. The hand that is closest to the adversary (e.g., just punched or blocked) performs the actual check, jam, or deflection, while the hand that is in chamber executes a technique designed to strike the opponent and/or control his limb. The arm-break block that I witnessed at the stadium was performed in this manner. The man who was attacked checked the incoming blow with one hand, pressed the limb to immobilize it for a split second, then struck hard enough with his other arm to hyperextend and damage his adversary's elbow.

The following is a more detailed description of the technique that I believe he used (he was too far away for me to be certain). We will assume the bad guy has thrown a right-handed punch as happened at the stadium. If it comes in from the left side, simply reverse which arm you use for each portion of the technique. You can block with either arm, of course, but you cannot get leverage against the joint to damage it if you pick the wrong side. If that should happen, the second movement would have to be altered into some other type of strike. This application has been broken down into three steps for clarity but you must perform it as one continuous movement to be effective on the street. Here's how it works:

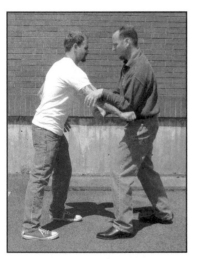

Check the incoming blow with your left hand, pulling it in and down.

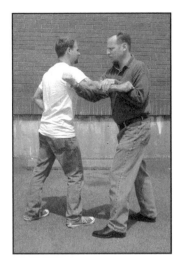

Control the limb by shooting your right hand up underneath as you would do for a normal left to right, outside chest block (*chudan uke*). Make sure your motion is out, across, then back in an elliptical movement rather than straight across.

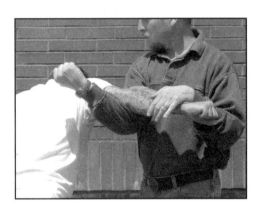

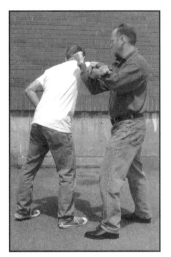

Third, set the block by dropping your weight and locking your stance, while pivoting your body with proper posture slightly to the right to hyperextend your opponent's elbow. In order to achieve maximum impact it is important to leverage with your whole body rather than just your arm, particularly if your adversary is bigger and/or stronger than you.

In practical reality you may or may not be able to damage the joint with this technique, yet done properly it, at minimum, will disrupt the follow-on blow, giving you a moment to counterattack. At best, it will dislocate your adversary's elbow in the same fashion I witnessed at the stadium, ending the fight.

Simple works best

When both your limbs are in play, you gain an inherent advantage in thwarting a bad guy's attack, typically making the most of a check/control or check/strike technique in doing so. While the resultant application could be an arm break, it is more common for it to be a strike. In this fashion, a head block (*jodan uke*), for example, can be performed with a deflection from the lead hand followed immediately by a forearm smash to the bad guy's head with the other arm. In an ambush situation, however, this type of thing does not always work. You might only be able to make contact with one limb before getting struck again, so I will focus on techniques that can strike or control using only the hand that makes first contact. If that first contact is sufficiently damaging, that will be all you will need to regain control of the encounter and set yourself up to escape to safety (possibly immediately but more likely after thumping the other guy at least once more in the process).

Shock blocks work because they are based upon simple body movements that can be performed under the effects of adrenaline. Since your heart rate can easily double in less than half a second during a sudden violent encounter, it is important to use straightforward techniques that will remain effective under extreme stress. Adrenaline can make you tougher, more resilient, and impervious to pain in combat, but it also degrades your motor skills, hand-eye coordination, precise tracking movements, and exact timing, making complicated techniques very challenging if not impossible to perform. Simple, straightforward applications, on the other hand, remain quite feasible, particularly those involving pre-programmed muscle reflex actions.

Duel in the sun

Following a time honored tradition of dueling (*kakidameshi*), *budoka* in ancient Okinawa routinely tested each other's fighting skills through actual combat. Like the feudal samurai before or the Old West gunfighter that would follow, the more famous the practitioner, the more often he was challenged to combat by those seeking fame. These fights were sometimes initiated by ambush and were often to the death, so such confrontations were not undertaken lightly.

According to legend, famed *Shuri-Te* karate master Itosu "Anko" Yasutsune traveled to the port city of Naha in the summer of 1856 to find relief from a particularly long period of heat and unbearable humidity. He found a large rock that provided some relief from the sun, settled down to enjoy the ocean breeze, and was about to doze off when he overheard several of the local villagers cracking jokes and disparaging Shuri karate.

Insulted by this banter, he decided to uphold the honor of his style by challenging the local champion, Naha-no-Tomoyose, to a duel. Making his way to the challenge area (*ude-kake-shi*), he made himself known to the crowd by quickly defeating three lesser practitioners in order to attract the local champion's attention.

When Tomoyose arrived on the scene, Itosu discovered to his chagrin that he faced a much larger, more powerfully built opponent. He realized that he would need to end the fight quickly or risk becoming overwhelmed by Tomoyose's superior size and strength. As the fighters began to circle each other, members of the crowd observed this disparity too, wagering at odds of ten to one against the challenger from Shuri. Tomoyose threw the first blow, a mighty lunge punch (*oi tsuki*). As Tomoyose's fist came screaming toward his head, Itosu shifted aside and blocked with a sword-hand technique (*shuto uke*), neatly breaking his adversary's arm. The crowd heard a loud snap, like the breaking of a branch, and the fight was over. This great victory, won through a basic block, solidified Itosu Yasutsune's reputation for all time.

Two types

There are two major types of shock blocks. I like to categorize them as torques and weight drops.

In physics, torque can be informally thought of as "rotational force," which is why I use this terminology even though it may not be precisely correct in the world of science. The rotation is important, working much like the crack of a whip. Examples of torquing techniques include things like rising head blocks (jodan uke) and inside forearm blocks (uchi uke).

Weight drops use the effect of gravity and bodyweight to amplify your striking energy, much like boxing legend Jack Dempsey demonstrated with his drop-step in the ring[3]. Examples of weight drops include palm-heel blocks (shotei uke), mountain blocks (yama uke), backhand blocks (ura uke), and press blocks (osae uke).

Some techniques combine both torque and weight drop. A good example is a down block (gedan uke) when performed as you drop into a low posture such as sumo stance (shiko dachi). We will go through each of the aforementioned examples in detail in a moment. A couple more principles need explanation first. When you perform a blocking movement you will either be opening your opponent up or closing him down.

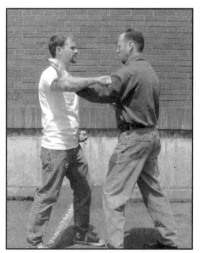

To open means that you are on the inside of your adversary's arms giving outward pressure. If you open the opponent, you expose his centerline, facilitating your attack yet leaving yourself more vulnerable to a counter threat. The centerline contains high-value targets such as the eyes, throat, solar plexus, and groin.

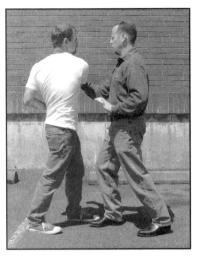

When you close your opponent, you are on the outside of the adversary's arm giving inward pressure to cut off his attack, leaving you comparatively safer. On the downside, there are fewer vital areas to aim for with your follow-on technique. You should still have access to decent targets such as the side of the head, floating ribs, kidneys, or knee. While the tactical situation will often force you to take whatever opening your opponent gives you, less experienced practitioners are usually best off closing for safety while more experienced practitioners may be best off opening to more quickly end the fight.

One last item before we get to the technique descriptions. To be most effective, contact must be an aggressive, powerful movement, much more like a strike than a block. It must cut off the attacker's technique before it gains too much speed and power, catching it as close to his body as possible. Even though I use the term "block," think "strike" as you perform these techniques.

Torque Blocks

Torque blocks use rotational force to shock your opponent, causing pain and disruption that may enable you to regain momentum and take control of

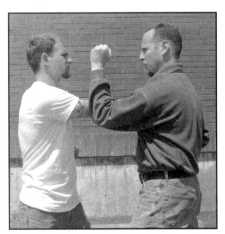

the fight. To get a feel for this, have a partner throw a half-speed punch at you. Hold your arm out and up, like you are a weightlifter flexing your biceps muscle, and then rotate your upper body to bring your arm straight across and cut off the blow with the inside of your forearm, hitting with the meaty part of your upper arm and then pushing through. This movement should readily deflect the punch but not hurt your partner.

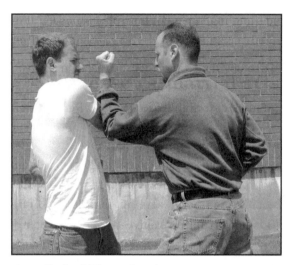

Now try it again a little differently. As soon as you make contact with the incoming punch, immediately rotate your arm inward so that the ulna bone (outside of the arm on the little finger side) makes contact with the incoming limb. Make this revolution quick and explosive, tensing your whole body as you complete the rotation. Even at half speed, this should be painful to your partner if you do it correctly.

Jodan uke (head block): This is one of the simplest torque blocks you can perform and one of the first taught in traditional karate schools, most likely because the initial blow in most fights is a strike to the head. Not only is the head a high-value, easily damaged target, but it is also a psychologically compelling one. Performed one-handed, *jodan uke* is very much like a punch.

To begin the technique, the leading arm closest to your opponent moves straight up, palm facing inward toward you. As your fist passes head height, your arm rotates over at an angle with your elbow pushing out such that your fist remains centered above your forehead. Finally, the forearm arm rotates outward, palm facing toward your opponent. This last movement generates most of the torque. You are now in a position to drive a punch into his midsection.

You can execute the head block as an opening or closing technique, of course, but I will show an opening technique in this example. If you move in on your adversary to close distance and your contact provides sufficient shock, you should be able to disrupt the integrity of his stance.

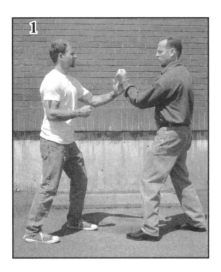
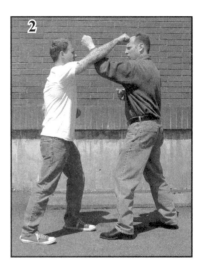

Physiologically this will force a small delay before his follow-on punch can come in with any force, as he will have to straighten, re-align his spine, and then throw the blow. During this momentary disruption, you will be able to counterattack. In this example the counter is a simple strike from the off hand.

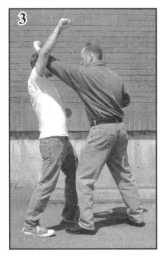
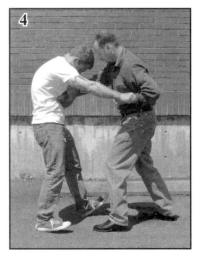

Uchi uke (inside forearm block): This is another great torque technique performed in the same fashion as the drill described at the beginning of this section. Because we can physiologically move outside-in (toward our centerline) faster than we can move inside-out (away from our center), it is naturally quick and very useful in a surprise attack. An instinctive follow-on is a sword-hand strike (shuto uchi). In some forms (kata), such as hookiyu and gekisai, this movement is combined with a simultaneous sweeping movement to extend the opponent's leg and stomping movement to damage his knee and/or ankle. While attacking both high and low at the same time in this fashion is much more effective than either technique alone, we will focus solely on the uchi uke for the moment.

Like the previously described jodan uke, you can perform uchi uke as an opening or closing technique. In this case, I will show a closing example. Once again, if you move in on your adversary to close distance and your contact provides sufficient shock, you should be able to cause a great deal of pain and disruption from this application. During this momentary disruption, you will be able to counterattack. In this example, the counter is a sword hand strike commonly seen in kata. While it may not be obvious while performing the kata, this application is typically an elbow strike (hiji ate) and then a shuto uchi, performed as one continuous movement. You simply lead with the elbow and the rest happens naturally.

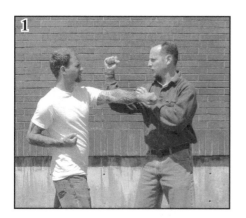 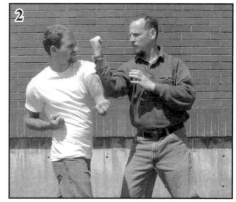

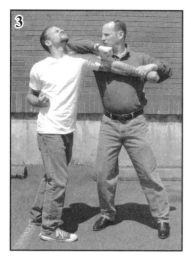 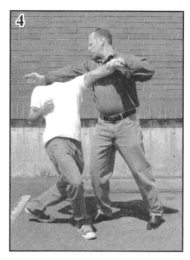

As mentioned previously, real fights are not static events. While a single application may certainly be able to end the confrontation, you simply cannot count on that happening every time. Consequently, combinations of techniques become very important. The aforementioned jodan uke and uchi uke make an excellent combination. It is natural, quick, and relatively easy to perform.

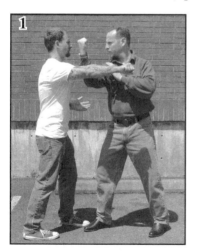 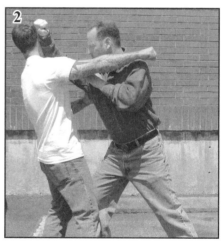

Above is an example of using the uchi uke to open an opponent with a follow-on jodan uke that, in effect, becomes a forearm smash. While shown in two steps it is performed as one continuous movement, using the bounce as the first block contacts your adversary's limb to facilitate a faster riposte with the second movement. Done properly, the first strike should be disruptive enough to give you time for the second which will hopefully end the fight, or at least put you on solid ground for doing so.

Weight-drop blocks   These blocks use gravity and bodyweight to amplify your striking energy. To be most effective, you will need to be extremely rigid at the moment of impact, connecting your arms to your body and aligning your spine so that all of your weight is transferred through your limb. If your body is loose, your arm will flex, diffusing much of your power.

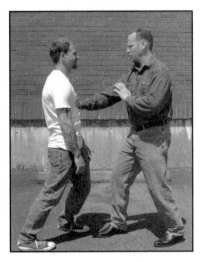

To get a feel for how this is done, place your hand against a partner's chest and push him backward using just your arm strength while your partner moderately resists (holding good stance, not punching or pushing back at you). Begin by standing close enough to your partner that you have plenty of room to extend your arm without having to step forward to move him.

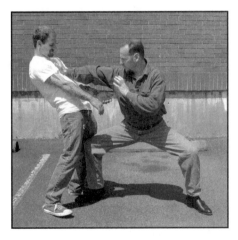

Now try the same thing again but put your whole body into it, dropping forward into a low posture such as sumo stance (shiko dachi). Be sure to move all your body as one unit so that your arm does not push all by itself. The power should come from your hips and bodyweight through your forward and downward movement. Done properly, you should notice that while pushing with your arm alone is good, pushing with your whole body is much, much better. Try it again with your partner strongly resisting (by stance alone) to get a good feel for the technique.

Shotei uke (palm-heel block): This is a basic but very effective weight-drop block.

It is performed often as a strike to the opponent's shoulder, pectoral muscle, or upper arm to cut short his attack, using a weight drop into shiko dachi for added emphasis. It can easily be followed-up by a blow from your off hand. In practical application, this technique must be performed with preemptive or simultaneous blocking. Used responsively, you will land your blow too late, almost assuredly getting hit on your way in by either the initial strike or its follow-on. When done properly, however, it can be very disruptive to your opponent. When you drop in place, throwing your arm out as your weight drops it can be extraordinarily fast, too. Body drops, arm shoots out. A good follow-on blow is to rotate your hips over into a forward stance (zenkutsu dachi) and punch with your other hand.

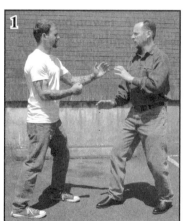
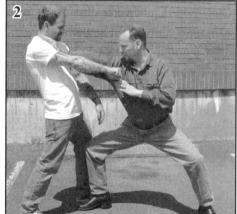
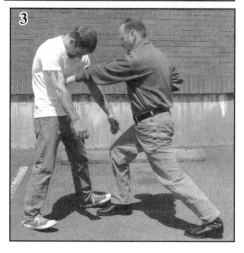

Yama uke (mountain block): This is an outstanding weight-drop block, somewhat safer than shotei uke since you automatically protect your head better in case you fail to connect with the incoming blow or otherwise mistime your technique. It is more offensive too, since it contains a simultaneous elbow strike. Furthermore, it has the additional benefit of working off your natural flinch reaction; many people automatically duck and cover their head when startled. In both cases, you are dropping to shiko dachi, a rather immobile stance, so you must not only be very close to your opponent but also strike swiftly and strongly so that you are not caught flat-footed.

On the street, yama uke can be very powerful when you drive forward into or through your opponent. You not only strike with your lead elbow but may also be able to connect against your adversary's legs or groin with your knee, depending on what type of stance he uses. Because you are so close, your rear arm (the one farthest away from the enemy) actually performs the defensive technique. If your lead elbow connects with the opponent's solar plexus, you might not even need a follow-on offensive technique. While he is gasping for air, you can escape to safety.

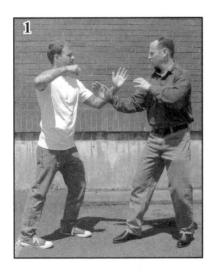 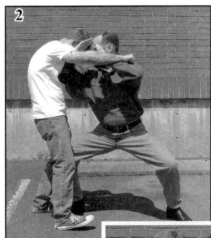

Ura uke (backhand block):   This is most effective when you shift off the line of your opponent's main force, striking downward at an angle. This technique is frequently performed in cat leg stance (neko ashi dachi) to facilitate a simultaneously swift evasion and body drop. Because this stance is very mobile, it is relatively easy to follow-up with an offensive technique. In practical application, it is important to think of this as a strike rather than a block. You are either evading the incoming blow or checking it with your off hand (or both) and then blasting down on the adversary's arm with the back of your wrist. Your weight drop into neko ashi dachi facilitates power for your technique and, as an added bonus, there are several pressure points along the arm that you may be lucky enough to hit.

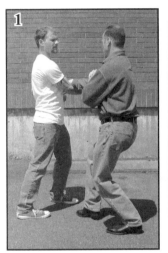
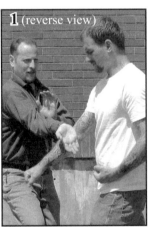

A common follow-on technique is an uppercut (age tsuki). This is often performed by striking again with your off hand to momentarily pin the opponent's arm while simultaneously shooting out the age tsuki with the hand that first blocked. If you shift forward into a more solid stance such as sanchin dachi (hourglass stance) your follow-on blow will have even more impact.

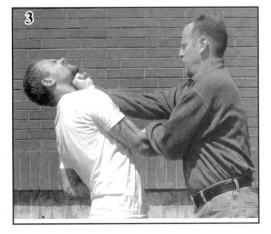

Osae uke (press block): This is generally considered an advanced weight-drop block. This is because the press is often executed with an internal weight drop where you lock into your stance, align your body, and lower your center of gravity, rather than as an external one where you drop in place by shifting to a lower posture. Even if you do drop into a low stance to take advantage of an easier-to-perform external weight drop, osae uke is executed by striking downward with your palm. This application requires more accuracy than blocks that utilize your whole arm. It is often performed in kata with a simultaneous palm-heel strike (shotei uchi). As one hand drops downward to perform the press, the other shoots out to strike your opponent.

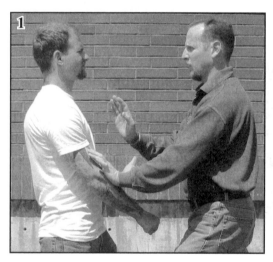 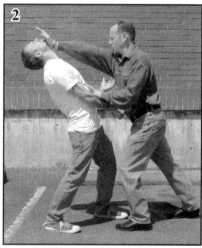

In practical application, osae uke is frequently used as an opening technique where you hold your ground, simultaneously cutting down the incoming attack and striking back with shotei uchi, a palm-heel strike. Like ura uke, you may be able to hit a pressure point on the arm for added affect. As the techniques finish, your body should be rigid with arms extended, one downward and one outward. Your shotei uchi strike may end up becoming a block if you have mistimed the application or your opponent turns out to be faster than you thought. Strike or block, either way it can keep you safe.

Torque/weight-drop blocks

Some defensive techniques use a combination of both torque and weight drop for added effect. The rotational energy of the arm movement is combined with the gravity/bodyweight drop to amplify your striking energy even further than can easily be done with either application alone. This becomes very important when working against a much larger or stronger opponent, or in cases where you wish to defend against a kick with an arm technique by striking rather than deflecting the adversary's energy with a sweep block (gedan barai uke) or hook block (sukui uke).

A good example of a combined torque/weight drop technique is the traditional down block (gedan uke). It works by both dropping into a low stance, such as shiko dachi, as well as driving the arm down with rotation at the point of impact. In this case, the torque is nearly identical to a jodan uke. You get more power if you use a push/pull technique (hikite) by simultaneously pulling your off hand into chamber.

This is a very common technique found in a plethora of kata yet it is much more powerful than many practitioners imagine. Use it offensively or defensively, as a strike or even as a throw. For example, your arm returning to chamber may have an opponent's hand or arm captured in it rather than just using hikite to increase your shocking force. To stick to the theme of shock blocks, however, I will demonstrate only an impact application, using gedan uke to defend against a kick.

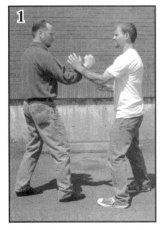
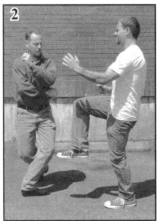
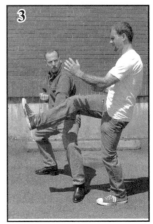

When performed in this fashion, you will frequently turn off-line away from your opponent's force and then strike his leg as it passes through the space where you just stood. You should tense your whole body on impact for best effect. This can be very powerful, indeed. In fact, I have nearly had my leg broken in this manner by someone who wasn't even trying to hit all that hard. Of course, he'd been doing this for more than 40 years so his light taps are stronger than most folk's full-strength strikes. Nevertheless, it's a robust technique, one that should not only shock the leg but also knock your adversary off balance if you do it right, facilitating your escape.

The faster you can dispatch your opponent in a real-life confrontation the safer you will be. To be most effective, your technique must simultaneously be able to keep you from getting hit while preventing your opponent from continuing his attack. That is why you should think of your defensive applications not as blocks, but rather as strikes. The Japanese word *uke* means receive rather than block; a significant difference in more than just the terminology. Solid, well-executed blocks can shock your opponent, causing damage and/or disruption that will let you regain control of a fight.

The two main methods of performing shock blocks utilize torque and/or weight drop to generate power, confound your opponent, and keep you safe. The applications I have described here represent a mere sampling of the various shock blocks found in *budo*. I encourage you to delve into your own martial art to find more. Tandem practice in the training hall (*dojo*) is a great way to internalize these techniques, facilitating your ability to use them effectively, should you ever need to do so, on the street.

---

*L*awrence Kane's biography appears in Chapter 6 "Makiwara: one blow on ekill." Thanks to Andy Orose for posing as the attacker and to Laura Vanderpool for her excellent photography.

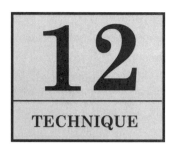

22 Ways to Kick 'Em High, Kick 'Em Low, Kick 'Em Hard, Kick 'Em Fast

By Alain Burrese

The advantages of kicking in a street fight include greater range, surprise, and power. The range from which you kick is farther from your opponent than the range from which you throw punches or grapple, so it can be a safer distance to launch your attack. Most strikes are thrown with the hands in street fights; therefore, throwing kicks can surprise your assailant. Additionally, your legs are more powerful than your arms, so kicks can generate greater force than other blows. To maximize these advantages, this chapter focuses on how to kick 'em high, kick 'em low, kick 'em hard, and kick 'em fast.

Kick 'em high

Many books and articles tell you never to kick high in a street fight and I've also recommended this to people. I've also joked that the only time you should kick someone in the head is when you put their head down at waist level or lower. That said I believe high kicks have their place in a person's self-defense skill set *if* the person wants to train sufficiently to use them.

A street fight in Korea

Once in Dongducheon, Korea, my buddy John kicked a guy in the head twice in one night. During the initial squaring off, John snapped a beautiful roundhouse kick into the guy's head. It didn't knock him out, but it did ring his bell. Immediately after that kick, two of the guy's friends jumped in to stop the fight, so I grabbed John, telling him it was enough. Unfortunately, the other guy didn't listen to his friends but rather shrugged them off and came toward John again.

While they again tried to hold him back and as I again told John to let it go, John snapped yet another roundhouse into the guy's head. This second kick ended the confrontation. His friends took him away and John and I left laughing as I commented on how nice his kicks were.

In this section, I discuss some of the pros and cons of kicking high for self-defense and share tips on making high kicks a viable tool. Make no mistake, you will have to train. A person can learn to throw a low kick in a brief time, but to become proficient enough to use them on the street requires serious gym time.

Advantages of a high kick

Kicking increases your range. Mid-level kicks increase your range more than high kicks, but even the high kicks affect range and distance.

Additional tools   High kicks provide you with additional techniques. Remember the saying, "If the only tool in your tool box is a hammer..." Increasing the number of tools, or options, available provides you with alternatives for the various situations you might face. You might never have the opportunity to throw a high kick in a self-defense situation, but if one does present itself, a high kick just might be the technique that saves the day.

Surprise and power   These are the advantages of all kicks, including high ones. A quick and powerful kick your opponent does not expect may end the confrontation with your adversary not knowing what hit him. Your legs are stronger than your arms, so why not use these powerful weapons to your greatest advantage.

Training to kick high improves your lower kicks   If you can kick high, most likely you can kick low very well. This does not mean you should only practice high kicks and low kicks will automatically be there. Kicking low is different from kicking high, and you must train for both. However, if you have the balance, flexibility and coordination to kick high, you will find that low kicks become easy to execute.

Disadvantages of high kicks

Let's look at some of their disadvantages and what we can do to minimize the risk involved with using these techniques. Make no mistake, the risks and disadvantages associated with high kicks outweigh the advantages, and that is why so many people tell you to never to kick above waist level in a street fight. However, with training, you can minimize the risks and have alternatives available to you during a fight.

Requires extra training time   The time it takes to become proficient at high kicks is considerably more than it takes to become proficient at low ones. So, if you want the most bang for your buck regarding training time, stick to the lower kicks. But if you want to put in hours of practice, you can make high kicks formidable weapons in your arsenal.

Require flexibility   High kicks take a greater degree of flexibility, which you increase through a proper stretching routine done consistently so its always there for you. If you can only kick high after a 20-minute warm-up, it won't do you much good in a parking lot facing a bad guy. In an actual self-defense situation, you must be able to execute your techniques, and that includes high kicks if they are to be part of your arsenal, without warming up or stretching.

Without stretching, your leg techniques will lack the power, speed, and accuracy. While your entire body should be stretched, there are certain parts that are critical to good kicks. These include the lower back, hamstrings, and the inside of the thigh or groin muscle.

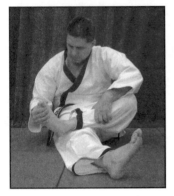

You should include ankle stretches since they support your body while kicking and landing during jump kicks. Injuries are prevented when your tendons and ligaments surrounding the ankles are kept flexible and warmed up during training.

I believe the stretching routines and principles outlined by Thomas Kurz in his book *Stretching Scientifically* can assist you in achieving the necessary flexibility for high kicks. Performing the dynamic stretching exercises Kurz describes and Mac Mierzejewski demonstrates in *Power High Kicks with No Warm-up* every morning as recommended, combined with other flexibility training and high kick training will enable you to execute kicks whenever needed. *Ultimate Flexibility: A Complete Guide to Stretching for Martial Arts* by Sang Kim, published by Turtle Press is another great source.

Besides dynamic stretching, these other methods might be beneficial:

- static stretching

- PNF stretching

- isometric stretching

- fascial stretching

- AI or active isolated stretching

- yoga can also complement martial arts or self-defense training.

Study and learn how to stretch and it will greatly improve your kicking skills.

Requires excellent balance Executing high kicks takes more balance than low kicks, and kicking in general takes more balance than keeping both feet on the ground. As we know, balance is crucial for fighting. Again, this aspect can be minimized through training. Work at improving your balance, but always remember that the higher your foot is from the ground, the less balance you have and the easier it is for your opponent to up-set you. While training minimizes this, it can't eliminate it. The good fighter recognizes weaknesses, trains to minimize them, and fights accordingly.

Restrictive clothing Kicking high can be limited by the clothing you wear. It's similar to the way in which wearing a chain around your neck can give your attacker something to choke you with, or wearing piercing-type jewelry can provide him something to rip out of your skin. Tight, restricting clothing limits your movements during a fight. Tight pants prevent you from kicking or they rip. Dress for the situations in which you might find yourself. Realize that clothing may limit the techniques you can use in a self-defense situation and defend yourself accordingly.

Pros and cons of high kicking at a glance

Pros

• Greater range
• Power
• Surprise

Cons

• Requires much practice to become proficient
• Requires more flexibility
• Requires more balance, especially on certain terrain
• Limited by clothing

Which kicks?

A fast powerful front kick is probably the easiest high kick to learn and it can be a formidable tool. Roundhouse kicks, sidekicks, hook kicks, crescent kicks, reverse crescent kicks, and back kicks above the waist can all be the deciding factors in a fight if executed properly with speed, power, and correct timing. In addition, you can effectively execute knee strikes above waist level, kicks that do not take as much training as some of the others. I do recommend you practice kicks under the guidance of an instructor or coach who trains in a kicking art. They can critique your kicks and provide valuable feedback on making them more effective.

The importance of chambering

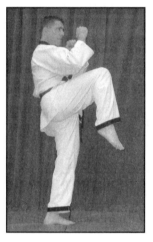

To execute a high front, side, or roundhouse kick, you must first raise the kicking knee and aim it at the target. This initial raising of the kicking knee is combined with a quarter pivot on the ball of the base foot to open the hips for the kick that is about to be executed. With the knee chambered high, you can then launch into a front, side or roundhouse kick at high targets.

While you can practice chambering your knee to increase the height of your front, side and roundhouse kicks, remember that when you are actually executing a kick, your knee is only in the chambered position for a split second. The kick becomes one fluid movement with your foot going from the ground to the target blindingly fast.

I may have gone against the grain by *not* telling you never to kick above the waist in a fight, but I believe high kicks have their place in training and in actual self-defense. The opportunities may not be plentiful, but when an opportunity does present itself, the person who trains in high kicking can take advantage of techniques that most people do not possess.

Kick 'em low

With all that I said about high kicks, low ones are still the bread and butter kicks for fighting, the primary ones used for self-defense. They are much easier to learn, they don't take near the practice to become functionally proficient at executing, and they are reliable against bigger, stronger opponents.

Many advantages

All of the advantages I mentioned when discussing high kicks are present with low kicks, but without the disadvantages. Sure, any kick requires more balance, but low kicks do not require the same as those above the waist. All kicks require training, but you don't need nearly the same training time to execute low kicks as you do the higher ones. Low kicks do not require the flexibility of high kicks, and clothing does not prohibit them as much as it can with higher ones. This is why low kicks are the bread and butter of kicks for self-defense and why so many people say only to kick low.

The best low kicks

The primary low kicks to practice are the:

- front kick
- side kick
- roundhouse
- scoop kick
- stomp

These five kicks are effective and they will take you a long ways toward defending yourself. If you don't know their basic elements, I recommend you learn from a qualified instructor or coach, with the possible supplementation of a good video or DVD, since that medium is more effective in teaching the entire motion than print. However, I will point out a few areas to consider when training or actually fighting with below-the-waist kicking techniques.

Chambering low kicks, or not

All five low kicks use a chamber. However, with modification, you can execute some without it. In general, chambering allows you to throw kicks that are more powerful, while kicking without the chamber tends to be quicker. Let's look at the scoop kick.

Scoop kick   Form the scoop by turning the toe end of your foot outward as you hit with the inside of your foot. Use this kick from a distance or while in a clinch.

To kick with a chamber, raise your knee and thrust downward, almost like a stomp, into your target. From behind a tall opponent, you can kick the back of his knee to drop him to your height to apply chokes or other restraining techniques. From your opponent's side or front, the scoop can be used to blast his knee into next week.

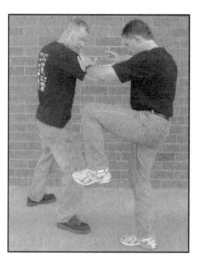 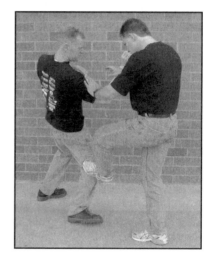

Without the chamber, the scoop moves in a rising motion, rather than a downward stomp. It can quickly go from the ground to the shin or knee to cause pain and set up another technique. Also, use it as a sweep to take away your opponent's balance; with proper timing, it will dump him to the ground. With practice, this fast technique can generate enough power to cripple your opponent and end the fight.

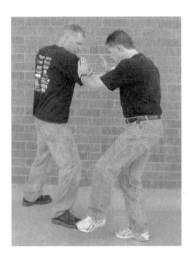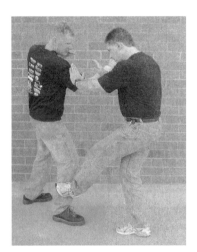

The groin and other precious targets

A good kick to the knee or stomp to the ankle can end a fight. Other good targets are the shins, instep, and groin. Do note that kicking the groin is not always as easy as it might seem due to many men's instinctive defenses to that area. However, if you do kick your attacker there, it is extremely effective in most instances. (There are people who wear groin protection on a regular basis, and others who can take groin shots and keep going.) These techniques are not lethal, but they can end an altercation and definitely aid your escape. No one will chase you with a blown out knee.

Roundhouse kick You have the same choices with the roundhouse kick as you do with the scoop. Without a chamber, the roundhouse can come smashing up from the ground into the outside of your opponent's leg creating a Charlie Horse by connecting with the peroneal nerve, making it difficult to stand, let alone chase you. Therefore, you want to practice the chambered versions of the kick for maximum power and the faster non-chambered version when it absolutely has to be there as quickly as possible. Both versions have their place in self-defense situations. Practice them.

Important point: With training, the fast non-chambered kicks will become more powerful and the chambered kicks will become faster, making your kicks an excellent means to defend yourself.

Blend your kicks with your upper body techniques

Since no single technique is perfect for every situation, you want to incorporate kicking techniques along with your hand and elbow techniques, especially using the high/low principle. As your opponent focuses on defending your hand strikes, he may be completely open for a low kick. A low kick directs his focus downward leaving him open for your palm-heel strike to his face. You need to be able to go from kicking to striking with your hands or elbows to kicking without a pause or loss of balance and motion. Slip, punch, kick. Move, kick, punch. Mix things up. Train this way and you will be ready to defend yourself with whatever technique the situation calls for.

Kick 'em hard

Kicking techniques can pack much more destructive power than hand strikes. Whether you are taking a guy's head off his shoulders, driving his testicles up between his lungs, or smashing his knee to smithereens, there is one thing to keep in mind: If you are going to kick someone, kick 'em hard. As mentioned, lifting your leg to execute a kick requires extreme balance and makes you momentarily vulnerable to certain counter attacks. With enough training, you minimize this risk. Keyword: minimize. Therefore, if you are going to assume the risk of using kicks, make the most of them by kicking with enough power not just to hurt your opponent but also to stop him devastatingly.

Kicking power and how to get it

Kicking techniques need driving and thrusting power to be effective. Without these attributes, your kicks will lack the needed power to crush and stop a menacing assailant. Many kicks rely heavily on explosive power generated from the upper legs and hips. You can take your kicks to a new level by increasing the strength and flexibility in the entire upper leg area, including the quadriceps (front thigh region), the hamstrings (back thigh region), and the adductor and abductor regions (inner and outer thigh). You must also strengthen the assisting and supporting muscles of the hips, gluteus maximus (buttocks), abdominal region, and lower back to maximize your kicking power.

Strength training   While this chapter is not about strength training it would be negligent to discuss kicking hard without addressing its importance. Many martial artists possess good technique but still lack power due to below-average leg strength. As mentioned above, there are numerous muscles working together during the execution of various kicks. The strengthening of those muscles will take your kicks to new levels.

For our purposes here, I will address a few exercises to include in your training. Please refer to other resources that specifically focus on strength training to learn how to perform properly any exercises with which you are not familiar.

Squats

First, the king of exercises: the squat. These build power, explosiveness and muscular size, and they will help increase power in all of your kicks as well as your overall strength, stability and balance. You can lose much of your kicking power if your balance is off. Squats strengthen your quadriceps, hamstrings, hips, gluteus maximus and your lower back, all while improving your kicks' thrusting and driving power.

Variations of the squat, include:

- front squats
- hack squats
- sissy squats
- single-leg squats
- jump squats

For variation and to increase intensity levels, exchange these in your routine periodically. Each works the muscles a bit differently and will increase your strength gains and promote more explosiveness in your techniques.

Leg extensions

The leg extension is an isolation movement that works the front thigh area, or quadriceps. Besides strengthening the quadriceps, leg extensions aid in strengthening the ligaments and tendons that connect the muscles that surround the knee. I don't need to emphasize how important it is to have this joint strong and stable for kicking success. Besides making your kicks stronger, strengthening this area will help hold your knee in place, thus preventing various joint and tendon injuries.

Leg extensions: good or bad?

Some experts believe that leg extensions are a potentially dangerous exercise because when only your shin is in motion, the exercise impacts the knee cap in such a way that it can damage the connective tissue and the ligaments supporting the joint. Should you have knee problems, skip this exercise. Likewise, if you have healthy knees but this exercise causes you pain.

Leg curls

It's important to have strong hamstrings to complement your quadriceps and add power to your kicks. These muscles work together to stabilize the knee; unbalanced muscular development may cause various injuries. Muscles work in pairs, and if one part of the pair becomes too strong in relation to the other, force output capability suffers. Your quadriceps are the prime movers (agonists) during kicking while your hamstrings are the antagonists. If you only train your quadriceps because they are the primary kicking muscles, your hamstrings become weak in proportion to your quads, and your power output declines.

Leg curls, standing and lying, isolate the hamstring muscles. (Check out Loren Christensen's *Solo Training 2* and *Solo Training DVD*, both published by YMAA Publication Center, for some tough hamstring exercises on a Swiss ball as well as core exercises mentioned below.)

Standing calf raise

While the calves are not specifically used in executing powerful kicks, they are important for moving quickly on your toes and the balls of your feet. Strong calves can give you bounce and spring in your kicking techniques, aid in quick footwork, jump kicks, and help your balance.

Do standing and seated calf raises with free weights and on any of several machines available in health clubs. They all stress the calf muscles a bit differently and you can easily work them into your workouts for variation.

Lunges

Lunges to the front, rear, and side not only help strengthen your muscles, but help stretch your legs as well. These can be done without weights or while holding a barbell across the shoulders or dumbbells in your hands. For safety, I recommend doing the versions holding dumbbells rather than those with the barbell. Lunge variations work the quadriceps, adductors, abductors, hip extensors, knee extensors, hip flexors, and gluteus maximus, depending on the direction of your lunge.

Plyometric jumps

Plyometric high jumps are an advanced exercise that adds explosive power to your kicks. Done properly, this exercise emphasizes all of the muscles of the leg, including the gluteus maximus and lower back. Variations of lower body plyometrics include:

* vertical jumps
* jumps between benches
* side-to-side hops
* lateral hops
* depth jumps

* kangaroo jumps
* jumping over objects
* single-leg hops
* single leg lateral hops

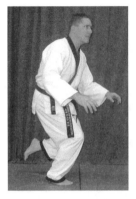

To do plyometric single-leg hops, start from a standing position with your left leg curled up behind you. Using your right leg, jump as high as you can and then drop into a half squat, less as you become fatigued. Without pause, explode back up with your right leg as high as you can, and then again drop back into a squat. Do 1 sets of 10 reps with each leg.

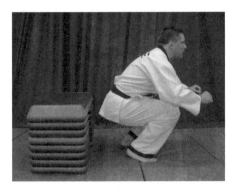

Do depth jumps by jumping off a bench (15 inches high for beginners, higher for advanced athletes) and land on the floor in a squat as pictured. Then, without hesitation, explode up as high as you can and drop back to the floor in a standing position. That is 1 rep. Step back up onto the bench and repeat. Do 1 set of 10 reps.

The secret with all of these exercises is to explode. Explode hard and 10 reps are all you can do.

Again, plyometric exercises are advanced so you should be in good shape before adding them to your strength program. Because of the high stress these exercises place on the body, you should use extreme caution when adding plyometric exercises to your routine. Do them no more than one or two times per week.

Training the Core

To become an excellent kicker you need powerful legs and you must strengthen your core, the stabilizing muscles of your abdomen and lower back. These muscles transmit forces from the lower extremities to the upper extremities (such as when you execute a correct punch starting from your toes), or from the upper body to the lower body (such as when you deliver a spin crescent kick). The core musculature also plays a significant role in stabilization during almost every movement.

Stabilizer muscles are those that anchor or immobilize one part of the body, allowing another part (usually the limbs) to exert force. The most important are those of the trunk – the abdominals and trunk extensors. Training the core completely includes exercises for the:

- trunk flexors (the rectus abdominous), such as crunches or hanging leg-raises.

- exercises for the trunk extensors (the erector spinea), such as back extensions and "good mornings."

- exercises for the side flexors (quadratus lumborum), such as dumbbell side bends.

- exercises for the flexor-rotators (the internal and external obliques), such as twisting crunches and their variations.

- exercises for the hip flexors (the illiopsoas, illiacus, and rectus femoris), such as sit ups, leg raises, and "flutter kicks."

There are many programs designed to strengthen the core muscles and I recommend using a variety of exercises including those with the large physio-balls or yoga, Swiss, and pilates balls, as well as medicine ball and partner training. Train your core to execute powerful kicking techniques.

Converting that newly developed power into your kicks

Once you strengthen your legs and core muscles, you're able to throw kicks that are more powerful. To do so, you need to convert that strength to the specific movements or techniques you have learned. One of the best ways to turn your gained strength into powerful kicks is through heavy bag and kick-shield training, hitting them at full power. Front kicks, roundhouse kicks, sidekicks, back kicks, scoop kicks, and stomps can be performed on heavy bags and kicking shields.

Note: The crescent kick should not be performed on a solid target due to the damage you will cause your knee.

Heavy bags and kicking shields allow you to throw full-power kicks into a target similar to an actual opponent. If you don't kick properly, and commit enough weight into the kick, you may knock yourself backward when your foot connects. You want to train properly with a heavy bag or shield before needing them for self-defense.

You don't have to go full bore every day for impact training to be beneficial. Like other forms of strength training, resist the urge to over train. Periodize strength training, heavy bag training, speed training, and accuracy and agility training throughout your workouts for maximum gains with minimum injuries. Periodization is simply "planned variation" of your training on a cyclic or "periodic" basis. You can vary your exercises, intensity, and volume to increase gains and prevent over training.

Kicking in the air is great, but you need to impact with something solid to use your techniques for self-defense. Heavy bag and kick-shield training helps you strengthen your kicks and give them devastating power needed to stop an altercation. You are not kicking to score points on the street; you are kicking to put your attacker out of the fight.

Kick 'em fast

Since your foot has to travel a lot farther than your hands when throwing high kicks, it is imperative that you include speed training in your workouts. You must be able to kick 'em fast if you want your kicks to be effective for self-defense. If your techniques don't land, they are not going to do you much good. Likewise, you must be fast enough to get out of the way or counter the techniques an attacker is throwing at you.

Speed components

There are several elements to speed and each is important when referring to how quickly you can get your foot from its starting point to the intended target. If you study speed more in depth, you can break it into several elements and get quite technical. I encourage more research into everything I'm writing about here. For simplicity, however, I'm only going to have you think about and train for two: reaction and movement.

Reaction time   First, you must develop quick reaction time. During a fight or an attack, openings for offense or defense might only be available for fractions of a second, so you need to possess the ability to react to such openings instantaneously. Your brain must recognize it, select the kick that can hit the target, and then send the message to the muscles that will launch the kick. Intense sparring assists in the recognition of targets and reacting to the openings, as well as other drills in which you react to a certain stimulus.

Reaction speed drill:

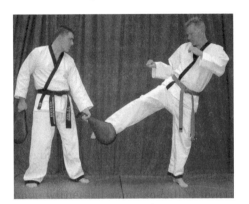 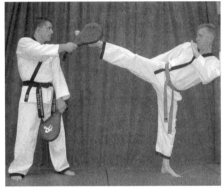

To develop my student's reaction speed, he must instantly kick the pad at whatever positions and height I move it. As he improves, I continue to present the target quickly but now I call out different kicks for him to use.

Movement speed   This refers to how fast your muscles can move your foot to its intended target. Part of movement speed is determined by your genetic makeup. All of us have both slow-twitch and fast-twitch muscle fibers. Your ratio of these fibers determines your potential for developing speed. Marathon runners tend to have a high proportion of slow-twitch fibers, while sprinters have a predominance of fast-twitch fibers. If you are lucky and have a predominance of fast-twitch fibers, you may become blindingly fast and be the next Bruce Lee. But if you don't, don't despair because you can improve upon what you have through exercise and training. In fact, the stretching and strength training already discussed can help increase your speed. Combine that with proper technique and form, along with specific speed drills, and you will be amazed at how fast you can move.

Incorporating speed drills into your training is essential. These should be performed when you are fresh and at your peak, not at the end of a long grueling workout. You should be using a periodization model for your workouts as mentioned in "Kick 'em hard," and speed training is one of the components that you schedule into it.

Movement speed drills:

Drill 1:

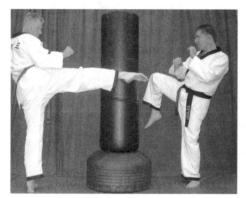 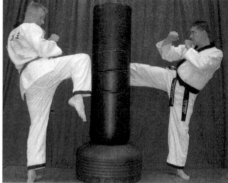

You and your partner face the heavy bag. Each of you kicks the bag in an alternating fashion as fast as you can.

Drill 2:

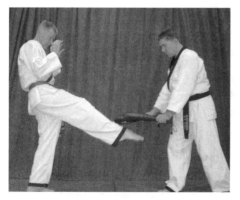 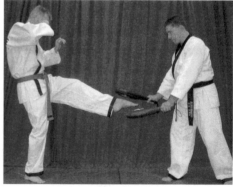

To develop quick footwork, your partner holds the kicking pads as you throw alternating kicks into them as quickly as you can.

Drill 3:

Your partner calls out various kicks for you to land on the heavy bag with minimum time between them. He calls them out increasingly faster as you get faster. To make the drill even harder, he calls out which leg for you to kick with and to where: "Left side kick stomach, right reverse crescent face, left back kick stomach," and so on.

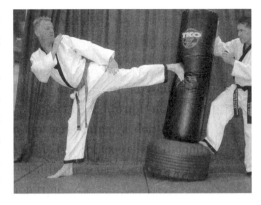

Drill 4:

Your partner holds a stopwatch to time you and count the number of kicks you land on the bag in 10, 20 or 30 second bursts. This great workout improves your speed and cardiovascular system.

Drill 5:

This time as your partner holds a stopwatch to time you in 10, 20 or 30-second bursts, he calls out which type of kick for you to land on the bag.

Kicking accuracy A fast powerful kick is mostly useless if you can't hit your target. You need to practice kicking with clap pads, hand-held double-sided pads that look a little like racquetball racquets and make a smacking sound when hit.

- Have a partner hold a pad for you. If you are just learning a kick, your partner will hold it stationary at a level that allows you to hit the target. As your skill and flexibility develop, your partner can raise the pads to create higher targets.

- To add difficulty to your drills, have your partner hold a pad in each hand and offer them as targets at various heights.

- Once stationary kicking becomes easy, you can move up and down the training floor as your partner offers the pads at various heights while you move both forward and backward while kicking.

- Finally, you can move around in a more realistic fashion with your partner offering various targets for you to kick. Your goal is to move quickly and to be able to respond from any position and angle with either leg, kicking precisely and accurately.

Sparring

No matter how well you can kick a stationary target or moving hand-held pads, there is no substitute for a live opponent who hits back. Sparring is important for kicking skills because it teaches balance, distance, and timing, all of them important factors when you need to kick 'em fast. While sparring is not the same as an actual fight, it can help you develop the skills needed for the street. Because some sport rules create bad habits for real fighting, I recommend sparring sessions that make the participants focus on self-defense basics as well as for whatever specific techniques they are training.

If you practice a martial art that teaches kicks, the information in this chapter will help you make those kicks more street effective. If you do not practice a formal martial art, I recommend learning basic kicks first while using the ideas presented in this chapter. Seeking out a qualified instructor to teach you how to kick is always the best way to learn. A qualified instructor or coach will be able to watch you move and provide feedback to correct your form and increase the effectiveness of your kicks. There are some excellent instructional DVDs out there than can teach an awful lot, but nothing beats having a good, live instructor.

Kicks are an excellent tool for the street, but only if you have learned them well and have trained hard. Include the ideas in this chapter in your training, and if you ever find yourself having to defend yourself, remember to kick em high, kick em low, kick em hard, and kick em fast.

Alain Burrese started training in Judo in 1982. Since then, he has trained in karate, taekwondo, boxing, qigong, and hapkido. He has lived and trained in South Korea where he continues to return to train with his hapkido instructors. He is the author of *Hard-Won Wisdom From the School of Hard Knocks: How to Avoid a Fight and Things To Do When You Can't or Don't Want To* and the instructional videos *Hapkido Hoshinsul: The Explosive Korean Art of Self-Defense and Streetfighting Essentials: Combining Western Boxing* and *Hapkido into an Unstoppable Self-Defense System*, all three available from Paladin Press. He served as a paratrooper and sniper instructor with the U.S. Army. He also worked as bouncer, security, and bodyguard, all of which add to the practical side of his instruction regarding real fights and violence.

Alain teaches self-defense and hapkido classes in Missoula, Montana, and travels to teach seminars on self-defense, hapkido, and the cane. His DVD set on the hapkido cane will soon be released by Paladin Press, and he is currently working on new DVD projects with both Paladin Press and Aiki Productions, as well as different writing projects. You can read articles and find out more about Alain's books, videos, and seminars at www.burese.com. You can also e-mail him at aburrese@aol.com.

Thanks to Todd Howie for posing and to Jay DeVore for his fantastic photography.

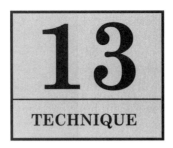

16 Techniques for Infighting

By Rory Miller

Bad things happen at close range. We're talking in-your-face, chest-to-chest, and halitosis range. With the exception of duels and friendly matches, most fights don't start and certainly don't finish at "bowing-in" range or in a place with lots of room to move.

Infighting is the ugliest range in which to fight. Things happen fast there. Distance is time, and with short distance you rarely, if ever, have time to block. It's complex: at infighting range strikes, kicks, locks, takedowns, clinches, trapping and strangles are all possible; so is biting. And it's scary - the human animal is conditioned to respond to an attack at this range as if a predator were attacking. Most people freeze.

There are few good infighters because it's hard to find training that covers all of the possibilities of the range. It's also rare to find a person who has the instinct to close with danger and has taken the time to get comfortable with fighting at a range that panics most others. The combination is devastating and intimidating.

Mutual recognition

Whenever I have a criminal about to go off in the jail system in which I work, I purposely step into his personal space. Almost everyone backs up, which gives me the psychological advantage. The ones who don't step back are the infighters. When they recognize the same tendency in me, they usually decide to talk because they know that if it goes bad, there is going to be a lot of pain to go around.

When a hug is more than a hug

Once when I was in booking, I heard a fresh arrestee yelling. Since kids will read this, I won't quote him exactly. Just know that it wasn't nice. He was swinging his arms around after being fingerprinted and the two officers assigned to the post were standing back, hoping he would cool off. I walked up and put my arm around his shoulders, smiled, and said, "Partner, you might want to rephrase that." He went white. He was being angry and expected fear in response, not a hug. That scared him.

Part of the skill of infighting is to have a thorough understanding of body mechanics and options. When I hugged the prisoner from that extremely close and seemingly vulnerable position, there were many options available to me. For example, my exposed ribs were at risk to his elbow. But by simply placing myself in contact with the leverage point at the back of his elbow, I prevented him from striking, unless he overtly drew his arm back, in which case my hip

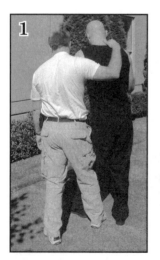 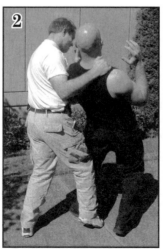

was placed for a slam to take him off balance or into a wall.

At the same time, my right hand could push or pull on his shoulder to disrupt his balance, pin his weight on one of his heels to immobilize him, or take him down.

My right, inner elbow was in position for a clothesline snap to the base of his skull, a dangerous but reliable fight ender. This is done by shooting the arm straight past the head as if you were punching high, allowing the inside of your elbow to impact the base of his skull. Here is another way to think of it: If you were to hold a belt loosely at each end, then suddenly pull your hands apart, the middle would snap straight with significant impact. Like the belt, the middle of your arm snaps with impact against the back of his head when you shoot your arm straight past it.

My right knee was set to pop his knee forward, either combined with the shoulder pull to dump him onto his back or to press down and force him to his knees.

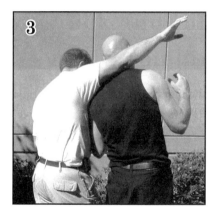 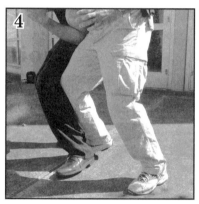

Not bad for a simple hug, huh?

There are four general things you can do at very close range: cause damage, disrupt balance, immobilize, or clear. If you're good, you can do them all simultaneously.

Cause damage

Striking at extremely close range is a special skill, and like any type of striking, it's based on timing, targeting, and power generation.

Although timing is one of the most complicated and fascinating skills in the martial arts, in real fights it's simple: You hit people when you can get away with it or you hit them when you have to.

When you can get away with it

If you can justify striking, then you should strike whenever and wherever you have an opportunity. His ribs are open, hit them. His knee is straight, pop it. You don't have time to create a layered game to get the perfect strike to the perfect target; you just do the best you can at the target that presents itself. We call that "recognizing gifts."

When you have to

You are taking damage, you hit the guy. He winds up to hit you, you hit him. You see the flash of steel that might be a knife at close range, hit him. He reaches under a jacket, you go for it. You don't idly take damage while waiting for an opportunity to strike "properly."

Targeting

The human body is a great big cat toy. As your skill at different kinds of movement grows, the available targets increase. The low, close-range fist targets include the liver, floating ribs, bladder, and groin. As you learn different ways to use your hands and arms, the pelvic gap (where the lower part of the pelvis isn't completely fused), pelvic arch (or pubic bone), and inguinal nerve (in the crease where the thigh joins the pelvis) become good low targets.

The head is a terrible target for the closed fist, but as you learn to strike with your head, there are interesting applications.

As you feel your own skull, the parts that feel like "corners" (above and outside the eye and, back from there, the length of the skull) are your weapons. Your targets are the flat places, such as the temple and jaw hinge. The nose is good, but there will be a lot of blood. The lower face might be more dangerous than it's worth - you will almost certainly break teeth and they will almost certainly tear your skin, resulting in blood-to-blood and saliva-to-blood contact. Remember, there are some nasty diseases out there.

Here is a basic list of targets that I teach my law enforcement students:

eyes	base of the skull
ears	throat, clavicle

solar plexus	liver
floating ribs	bladder
groin	arch of the foot
fingers	bones in the back of the hands.

peroneal nerve on the outside lower portion of the thigh

As I said, the human body is just one big cat toy.

Generating power

While speed is a huge component of power, there generally isn't sufficient space at close range to generate enough of it. However, there are several other ways to build it. My favorites can be divided into muscle-based power (rotation, lift and whip) and gravity based power (drop, bounce and wave action).

Muscle-based power All that a karate sensei tells you about generating power is true: putting your hips into a strike will make you hit harder. Snapping your offside hand back will make you hit harder. At close range, using a wider and deeper stance will make you hit harder. If you don't want to listen to a karate guy, you should know that Jack Dempsey gave almost the same advice in his classic *Championship Fighting: Explosive Punching and Aggressive Defense.*"

These elements are the key to a close-range power strike, whether with elbows, fist or open hands. I'm not a big guy, but I've twice broken ribs through armor. I did it once on a man wearing entry armor (the heavier armor that a tactical team wears when they are going through a door or dealing with a riot), and once to an officer wearing a bullet resistant vest in a session in which we were training in our duty equipment. I was even wearing boxing gloves.

To generate power in a linear strike, your rear heel digs into the ground at impact. If the timing is right and slop is removed from the physical structure, the power of a kick can be generated through your fist. Slop means all the little shock absorbers and rotational inefficiencies that can creep into a technique.

Lift can be added to either a circular or linear strike when the angle of the strike is somewhat upward. Drop your weight slightly and surge upwards with your legs. This uses the threat's own weight as a basing surface for the strike. (See "My plug for traditional stances.")

Basing

You can improve almost any strike, especially to a soft surface, by removing the threat's ability to move with the force. A target pinned against the wall or lying flat to the floor will absorb the entire force of an elbow strike or knee drop. Striking joints is rarely effective unless the limb is pinned or held. A good infighter transitions between strikes and grabs, using the grabs to create a base for a second strike. For example:

- Execute a slap to an opponent's jaw hinge or ear. From there, transition to a hair grab and pull his head into a punch from your other fist.

- Use the ground as a base point by directing strikes downward. A knee drop on a downed threat is one example, but even a downward elbow strike to the collarbone uses the same principle, with the threat's leg strength providing part of the power of your blow.

- Use gravity as a base by striking upward so that the threat's own weight acts as a damage absorber. An uppercut to the solar plexus can do more damage than a straight punch because the threat's mass moves less and thus dissipates the power less. In essence, it's using the opponent's weight as the tamping for an explosive charge

- When striking a hard surface, such as the head, I prefer to "semi-base." This means that I strike the head or I simply strike toward the head to draw a flinch from the person when there is a hard object positioned an inch or so behind him. The threat's flinch response will slam his head into a doorjamb or a corner of a building harder than I can probably hit with my fist.

Whip actions use a flexible motion of the limbs to deliver a stunning impact. It's easier to demonstrate at longer range with a throwing action, but the same principle, with practice, can be used at contact range.

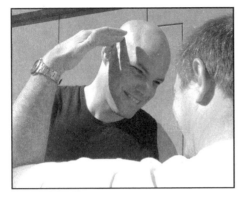
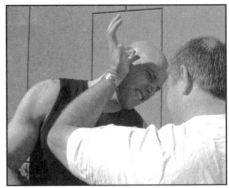

Whip action break at wrist...

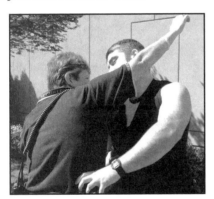
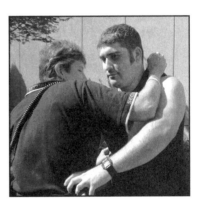

...and clothesline snap with elbow)

Gravity-based power   This is the big equalizer for small people.

Drop: Dropping your weight into the attack is simple: you suddenly take all the weight off the nearest foot to the threat and then fall, not step, into the technique. Falling is one of our few innate fears. When combined with years of training on the importance of keeping your balance, falling on purpose, sometimes called a drop-step, is one of the most difficult skills to acquire. But it is valuable and requires commitment... and infighting is definitely the time for commitment.

Bouncing: Bone bounces while muscle flops down and lays there. The key to a gymnast's handspring, for example, is to use the bounce of bone, not the flop or strength of muscle. A gymnast's arms are straight when he hits the ground and then his body weight bounces up and over. This idea is central to many so-called "internal" power martial arts systems. Basically, you suddenly drop your weight onto a leg that is almost locked to get the power of a drop step, but in an upward direction

Wave: The wave action is slightly slower but easier to understand. A crashing wave rises over the beach and then falls onto it; a surging wave gathers underneath and rises up. To duplicate a crashing wave, raise your center of gravity in a semi-circle as you move slightly toward the target and then let the power fall. To surge, drop your weight while sliding in, loading the muscles in your leg, and then lift upward as described above.

My plug for traditional stances

The traditional stances taught in most karate classes are fantastic examples of using gravity power. I don't usually like the way I see them taught, as there's no justification for staying in a low stance for any length of time. However, when you suddenly drop your weight, whether to strike, lock, or yank a threat off his feet, you land in one of several of these familiar stances. Additionally, each of these stances flexes the hips or legs ballistically to build explosive power for a rising attack. So, by dropping into a solid traditional stance, you generate a powerful downward attack, and then you generate a powerful rising attack when leaving the stance.

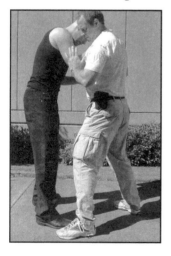

Use your left palm to clear a space by parrying his arm at his elbow leverage point.

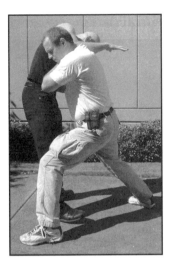

Drop your weight into a front stance as you simultaneous slam your right elbow into his liver.

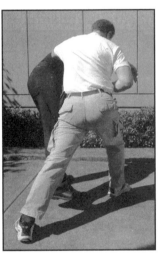

Your bent left leg then explodes into a hard pivot to your right into a front stance, simultaneous with a push or strike that knocks the threat away.

This just scratches the surface of power generation but here are two critical elements that martial artists often forget in real fights:

- Use a tool. The best technique for generating power is to use a tool from your surroundings: a stick, phone, book, or a cue ball in a sock.

- Don't forget the environment. Slamming the threat into the corner of a table will do more damage than your fist will. Learn to exploit opportunities.

Throughout this section, I've used striking as an easy example. The same principles that generate power for striking will also turn a lock into a decisive break or a takedown into a solid slam.

Disrupt balance

It's sometimes just as useful in a fight to disrupt balance as it is to do damage. Most systems of power generation require solid contact with the ground. When you deny the threat contact, you deny him power. It's difficult for him to hit you at all when he is falling or being moved involuntarily. A sudden sensation of falling especially freezes his mind and disrupts his timing.

Balance basics

Your feet create a base no matter how you stand. For example, the base in a natural stance is a rough square of four lines, the outside edges of each foot, the toe of right foot to the toe of left foot, and heel to heel.

Your center of gravity (COG) is located at about belt-buckle level between your navel and your spine, a point where your body balances in all directions. If your COG leaves your base, you lose your balance. If you are not able to recover, you fall.

You can disrupt balance by forcing or influencing the COG to leave the base or by changing the shape of the base. Six ways to do that are:

1) **Maximize leverage** Pressure on the chin shifts the center of gravity with less effort than pressure on the chest or pressure at waist level.

2) **Apply force upwards** Lifting up on the chin, armpit, elbow, or any other point will more efficiently move the COG (and may break connection with the ground) than horizontal pressure. Pressure downward sets the threat more solidly into his stance.

3) **Use spirals** Upward twisting force is harder to resist than simple upward force.

4) Work against the spine Since the spine is less flexible to the rear than it is to the front, leverage action on the spine backwards will be harder to duck or slip than pressure to the front. As already mentioned, the spine is also vulnerable to twisting and lifting spirals.

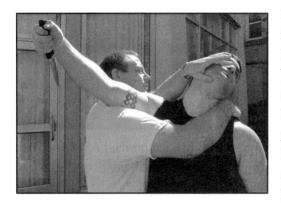

In this situation, you're applying force upwards against his jaw leverage point. By bending him backwards, you are forcing him against the natural direction of his spine. By turning his head, you are applying a spiral twist. Note that by trapping his elbow at the leverage point you prevent him from stabbing you.

5) Use leverage points Pressure on the back of the elbow, base of the nasal bone, chin, and jaw are more effective than other points for moving a body. This is because you're pitting your strong muscles against the threat's relatively weak muscle groups at a point of great leverage.

6) Take advantage of "gifts" If the threat surges or moves hard, he will shift his COG closer toward an edge of his base. Fine. Help him along.

When changing the base, you can:

1) break the threat's connection with the ground.

2) move an edge of the base so that the COG is outside of it.

3) destroy the structure that keeps the COG above the base.

Breaking ground connection You can do this with a throw, by getting your COG under the threat's COG, and lifting him. Or do it with a hard foot sweep, where you "chop" out his base.

Move edge of base When a threat isn't moving, you can move the edge of his base with a light sweep against only one of his feet. A moving threat is always in transition as his COG moves from base to base to base. (Walking is a type of controlled falling forward, where one foot leaves the ground, thus placing all of the walker's weight directly over his remaining foot. As the walker's COG leaves that tiny base, his other foot moves forward to catch the weight.) To unbalance a moving threat, you must remove the foot (sweep it) before it can catch the COG.

Destroy the structure This implies popping the threat's knee to the rear or to either side of its natural motion, an action that can be crippling. To simply unbalance him, pop your knee into the back of his, reliably forcing him to kneel as he faces away from you. This is a prime position, as it's easier to neutralize people from behind.

Stacking: Combine as many of these principles as you can into each application. Instead of just manipulating a threat's COG or just altering his base, do both simultaneously to be twice as effective. The combination is greater than the sum of its parts.

Immobilize

You can prevent the threat from moving or striking using the concepts described in the "Fighting the core" sidebar and you can control the amount of damage he can do by controlling his space. At close range, there is a lot of body contact, which you can use to your advantage by smothering and dragging his attacks.

The classic boxer's clinch is an attempt to smother incoming attacks. Most fighters need distance to build enough speed for their strikes to be effective. If you press your body directly against a fist or elbow and "ride" it, it does no damage. When infighting with an elbow striker, I prefer to get the leverage point at the back of his elbow pressed against my neck. It not only neutralizes one of his best weapons, it ties up an entire limb without sacrificing any of mine. It also exposes his ribs on the same side as the arm I'm controlling.

Fighting the core

Since all parts of the human body are attached, with skill you can affect one part of the threat's body by applying pressure to another. The key is to understand the connection between the pelvis and shoulder girdle through the spine.

If you lay your weight on the threat's right shoulder, he can't lift his right foot. If you put weight on his right shoulder while forcing it forward off his base and slightly to his left, he can lift his left foot but he can't kick with it to the front. Also, his punches will have little or no power.

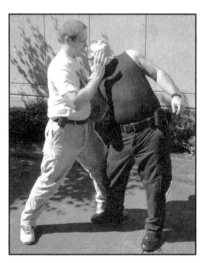

To effectively paralyze the threat, pull down on the threat's collar, hand, or the crook of his bent elbow, and

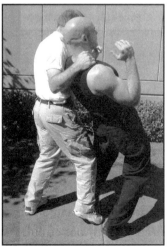

aim them at a spot between his heels and slightly behind him.

Push your knee into the back of the threat's left knee to abort a punch with his right hand.

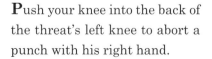

Three clinches

There are different clinches for different purposes. As mentioned above, the classic boxer's clinch is a defensive one, a combination of smothering and dragging that prevents the threat's fist from doing damage.

In contrast, a muay Thai fighter clinches to gain control of a prime target area, to clear space for his knees strikes, and to add damage to the strikes by a two-way action: pulling with his hands and striking with his knee.

A Tokugawa era (1603– 1867 Japan) jujutsu clinch serves a different primary purpose: Both arms are held in such a way as to prevent the opponent from drawing weapons from his belt or from yours.

Three different clinches for three entirely different reasons.

Dragging attack

This is the simple act of keeping one of your limbs on the threat's attacking limbs so that he must strike against your weight and resistance. Simply collapsing your arm into the crook of the threat's elbow and leaving it there doesn't block his limb, but it does prevent him from building up force to hurt you. You can then follow with anything you want, such as a chin push to twist his head away.

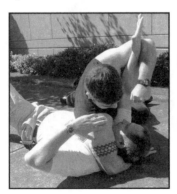 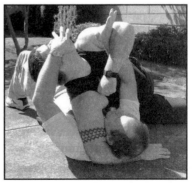

Spine Immobilizing This is used to freeze targets so that they are easier to hit and thus vulnerable to more damage.

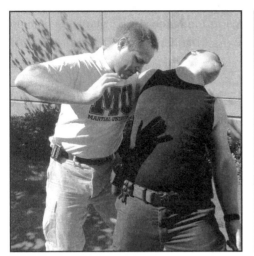 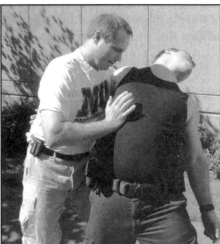

From a position with your chest against the threat's right side your left hand slips up behind his head and grips his hair. Drawing his hair back and downward not only pins him on his heels, but also exposes his throat and floating ribs. In fact, the position flexes his ribs outward so that they break more easily.

Clearing

If you can control space and time, you win. Clearing and immobilization are the critical skills for controlling space at close range. In the section "Immobilize," we talked about taking his space away. Now let's talk about creating space for you.

You clear space for yourself by either:

1) moving his body.
2) moving a part of his body.
3) or moving your own body.

Moving the threat's body

While many of the circular blocking actions taught in traditional striking styles are far too slow and obvious, they are perfect for clearing.

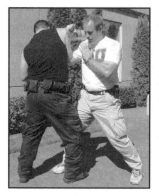 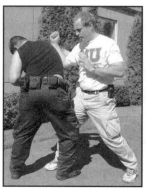 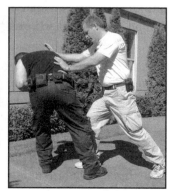

At extremely close range, the circular block motion comes up and under the threat's arm and exposes the floating ribs. With almost no modification, it pushes the threat slightly off balance and immobilizes him in place, a single action that allows for several follow-up options.

Moving your body

You do this by creating enough space to generate speed for striking without having to create distance. This was done in several of the earlier examples for hand strikes, such as pulling the hair to expose the ribs. The knee pop described above puts the threat in front of you and leaves you plenty of room to strike. However, kicking is a more challenging example, and more surprising for the threat.

Generally, kicks are the most range-dependant of all attacks, ruined when someone steps into them or away from them. Making space to kick at close range requires a fresh look at how to chamber and the available targets.

Targets will be lower and closer, and speed and power will come from a high or a long chamber. For example, the back of the knee is an excellent target for a stomp kick, even when you're in contact range and facing the threat.

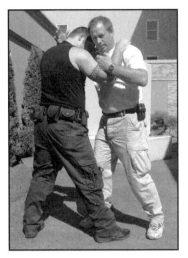 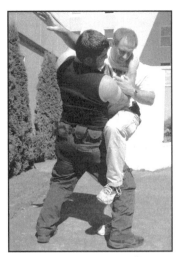

Maintain your grip on the threat, raise your knee, and slam your foot down into the target zone.

The lead-leg rear kick is more impressive. Even with poor to average flexibility, you can still deliver the kick at the threats' knee level while in a clinch. With good flexibility, you can deliver it to his solar plexus or floating ribs while looking in his eyes at hugging range.

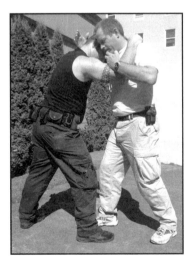 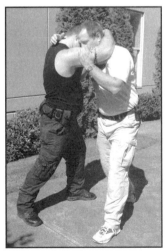

For a right leg kick, your right foot is slightly forward in the clinch.

Rock your left hip back to clear space...

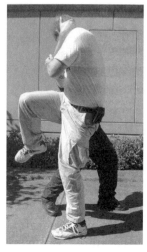

... and fire your right knee as far to your left as possible and as high as possible.

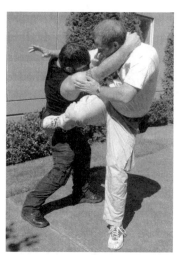

When it gets to the end of your flexibility, use the bounce in your tendons to fire it into the target.

Infighting isn't just a list of skills. The breadth of infighting skill is in knowing how to damage, how to take down, how to clinch, how to lock and strangle, how to strike, when to bite... many, many separate skills. The depth of infighting skill is the ability to do them simultaneously to strike, throw, and lock as a single action. It's largely a matter of practice, practicing until you no longer need to think about how they twist or fall, as you won't have much time to think at all under the stress of a real fight.

It's also a matter of heart. Fighting at this range is savage. I'm flippant about it in these pages, but when it goes bad at close range, someone is going to get hurt. Most people panic; they just freeze. Predators know this and try to ambush from this range. You have to be ready.

Practice.

*R*ory **Miller**'s biography appears in Chapter 4 "10 concepts to adapt your training to the street."

Many thanks to Jordan Wiley, Sally Harlow, and Luke Heckathorn for their work in front of the camera, and to Kamila Z. Miller for her fine photography.

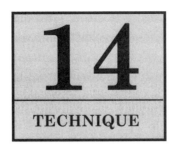

14 Hand-to-Hand Combat techniques: A Philosophical Look

By Richard Dimitri

How does one prepare for hand-to-hand combat (HTHC)? What is important? First, you must understand the way of the warrior, the way of death. It's elaborated on in the first chapters of Miyamoto Musahi's *The Book of Five Rings.* According to Musashi, a warrior is one who accepts his fate and sees himself as being already dead before entering combat. He has to accept this fact to perform at his peak.

Bruce Lee also said something to the extent of: If a man bruises you, break his bones; if he breaks your bones, tear his limbs off; if he tears your limbs off, take his life. Lay your life before your enemy.

How true. How can you do what you have to when you're too busy worrying about the consequences? If your mind is cluttered with thoughts prior to and during HTHC, then you're not concentrating on the moment at hand. HTHC is the most intense activity a human being can engage in.

It's about accomplishing what you need to accomplish to live another day; it's not a collection of moves in a catalogue that you memorize so as to bring them into play on cue like Pavlov's dog. To survive as intact as possible, you primarily need to reevaluate your belief system for one that is congruous to your objectives of survival. You need the proper mindset, a system of values and ethics not warped by some fancy and ludicrous perception given to you by individuals who have never "been there." Whoever engages you in real HTHC most often does not embrace your code of honor. We are not talking about two samurais getting into an epic battle at sunrise on some mountaintop.

Do you value human life as a general principle or do you value the life of individuals? Let me elaborate. We respect the life of humans but do not automatically apply this respect to anything that walks on two feet. Pedophiles, rapists, drug dealers, murderers and people who generally prey on the weak... well, they get much less respect than a cockroach deserves.

Your right to self-defense

The unwritten moral waiver prior to HTHC states that when someone chooses you as a victim, he is basically saying this: "I have chosen to attack you. Therefore, I accept the fact that I may sustain massive trauma because I am aware that you will do anything and everything inhumanly possible to save your life, and I accept and endorse the responsibility of what may happen to me during the course of this altercation."

Understanding this, you have the right to defend yourself at all costs. The individual before you is aware of theses consequences.

Defense against a rear choke

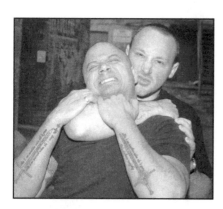

When you're attacked from behind, you reflexively grab the assailant's arm.

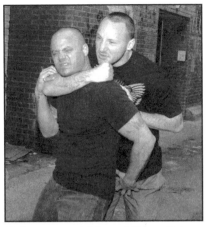

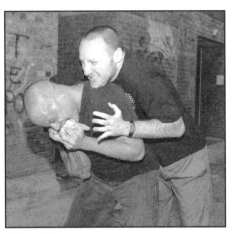

Side step quickly, while striking and grabbing the attacker's groin simultaneously.

Bite his arm

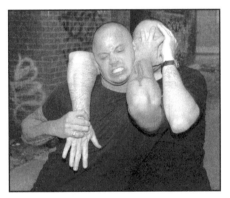

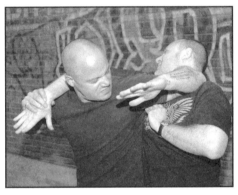

As the attacker continues to struggle, grabs one of his arms and claw his face

Elbow his face.

Finish him with a headbutt.

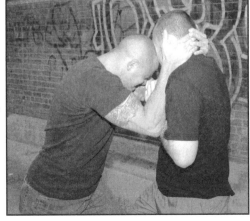

Your focus is not to find out if the sociopath has had a troubled childhood or if he is a victim of society. Your focus is to live, to survive. Any other thoughts during a violent confrontation will only prevent you from doing what you have to do to live another day.

It's not to say that every single fight ends up in a death, but stuff happens. Consider this. Years ago, during a July 4 weekend, a fight between two young men erupted in a park next to a large bonfire. The confrontation started with the traditional shoving match, but during the ensuing fight one of the participants shoved the other. The one shoved tripped, lost his footing, fell into the bonfire, and died. The one who shoved him didn't mean to kill him, but stuff happens, and because it happens, you must have all angles covered to deal with it.

Real combat is ugly

Hand-to-hand combat is probably one of the ugliest things you will ever encounter. There is no nobility or glory and it's not gratifying or valorizing. In the worst case scenarios, you feel horrible. You have to deal with the victim (what is left of him), your injuries, your adrenaline withdrawal, witnesses, cops, courts, and your spouse. Maybe you will have a little guilt, maybe a lot. Better to feel guilty than be on life support or on open display at your funeral.

The Shredder™

The Shredder is a close-quarter conceptual tool designed to shift the predatory/prey instinct and bypass the startle to flinch mechanism enabling anyone of any size or strength to successfully defend himself without prior training.

In short, The Shredder is a barrage of short, gross motor tools applied in succession on a quarter beat. It comprises many different tools such as knees, elbows, palm strikes, forearm shaves, strikes, claws, ripping, tearing, biting, spitting, and so on.

It is not a set of moves or memorized techniques but rather a spontaneous assault of gross motor tools launched on a quarter beat, attacking vital areas and making it near impossible for the "opponent" to intercept or stop once it's been properly launched. The Shredder is something people have been doing since the dawn of man when faced with threat of extreme violence. It's based on simple natural movements and is a concept that is behaviorally and scientifically rooted.

Self-defense using The Shred and an improvised weapon

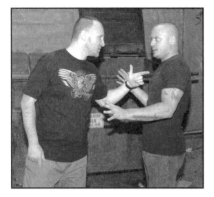

The assailant woofs in your face. Maintain a passive stance and try to diffuse the situation.

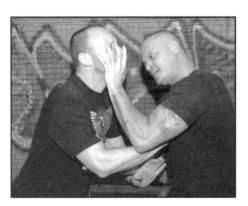

Since your hands are already up, you can easily intercept his attack by jamming his arm and then launching a shred to his face.

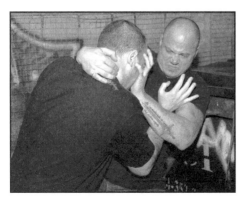

Continue to shred his face as you maneuver him off centerline to inflict maximum damage to him while minimizing it to you.

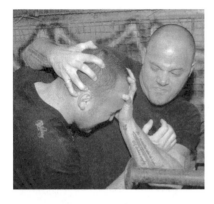

During the struggle, you see a garbage bin you can use as an improvised weapon. You maneuver him in position.

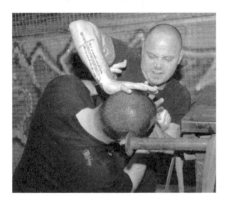

When the moment is right, slam that attacker's head into the bin. Be justified as this is a severe move.

Strategies and tactics

How do you develop the mental and emotional arsenal to be able to navigate through the chaos and mayhem?

Plan for it

You need tactical awareness and strategy. Tactics will get you out of trouble, not your jump spinning back kick and lunge punch combination. Tactics are simply what you can do with what you have at a given moment based on a previously thought out plan. Strategy is the overview; tactics are the immediate manifestations of strategy. Your tactics will have to be established in a blink of an eye and implemented in half that time based on your previously thought out strategies. Therefore, being proactive and thinking out a strategy for any given situation will tactically enhance your chances of survival.

Someone once said that fighting is like chess at 100 mph with muscles. He who is ahead of the game, wins. You have to take into consideration all of the variables we talked about earlier. Consider the terrain of the engagement, the possibility of artillery, multiple adversaries, and any bystander who has the potential of becoming an active participant. This data must be analyzed faster than the fastest computer and then it has to be acted upon accordingly. No room for mistakes. Mistakes can lead to a world of hurt, even a fatality. HTHC is 60 percent psychological, 25 percent emotional and only 15 percent physical. Anyone can learn how to kick, punch, or apply a choke, but how do you piece it together when reality slaps you in the face? The answer is options and strategy.

Skill in all ranges

The only way to implement a strategy of your choosing is to be versed in the discipline of fighting in all ranges. Being able to flow fluidly from one range to the next at any time during a high-stress situation is essential to your survival. The ranges of HTHC are as follows:

- Lunging range, where you can't land a kick but with a knife and a forward lunge you could give your opponent a new orifice.

- Kicking range, the second longest range in which you can only logically throw a kick

- Boxing/punching range, where you can land any punch in your arsenal.

- Trapping/close-quarter-combat range, where most fights start.

- Grappling range, standing or on the ground.

- Ground-fighting range, where most fights go when your close-quarter-combat is lacking.

Sub-ranges When integrating the ranges together you will notice that you can use tools from another range in the particular one you're in. For example, when in the boxing/punching range you have access to certain kicks from the kicking range and strikes from the trapping range. The nucleus is the mother range; everything flowing from it that doesn't belong to the nucleus is a sub-range.

Self-defense in multiple ranges

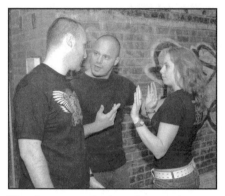

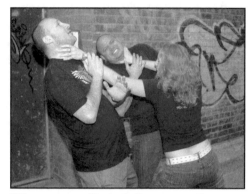

You have unwisely taken a shortcut through an alley when two thugs block your path. You try to defuse their threats and intimidation.

When your efforts fail, you continue talking to distract them. Shoot your hands from under their fields of vision and strike their throats.

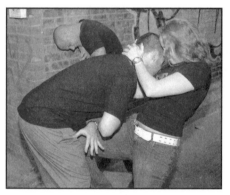

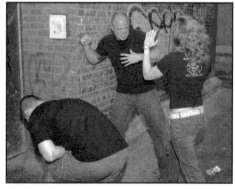

Grab the closest attacker and hit him with a solid knee strike as the man struggles to catch his breath from the initial throat strike.

As he crumbles, the other attacker somewhat recuperates and swings a right haymaker at you.

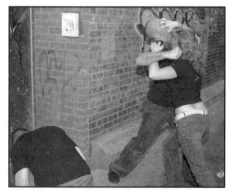

Jam his attack and shred his face.

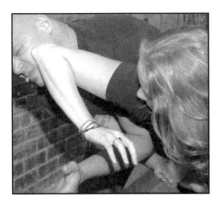

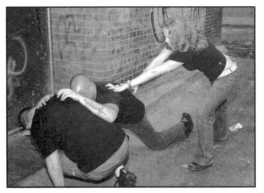

From the facial rake, fold your arm into an elbow smash. This makes your blow almost impossible to intercept.

Push the injured attacker into his injured buddy and run quickly out of the alley.

Weapons

The best way to understand a weapon is to know how to kill with it. Someone not qualified to instruct knife fighting is not qualified to teach knife defense. We have witnessed some so-called martial arts experts teach the most ridiculous defensive knife fighting techniques to their students, techniques that would get them killed. These so called "masters" have no social responsibilities whatsoever. It's also painfully obvious that they have never been in or witnessed a real fight.

Improvised weapons can be anything from a ballpoint pen to a pool ball to a refrigerator door. The book *Cheap Shots Ambushes and other Lessons* by Marc Mac Young (highly recommended for it's street psychology), tells a story of a guy who would always stand near a pool table in a bar before a fight would break out. He would put his buck in, get a rack of balls, and then wait for anyone to come near him. When someone did, he would whip a ball into the person's chest. Darts are also a good resourceful weapon, as are broomsticks, and pool sticks.

Your ability to deal with variables can be cultivated through regular realistic training. A responsible instructor or coach will constantly force his trainees to adapt to variations in drill format and create circumstances where trainees will have to go safely beyond their physical and emotional limitations. For example: Applying a hold on a willing partner in class is one thing but that same hold can dramatically fail *after* you have run for your life for two miles and then tried to do it on an opponent who doesn't share the same enthusiasm as your partner in class. Bottom line: You're training to save your life, which on its own is the ultimate stress management challenge.

Four principles of combat

1. Fear management
2. Understanding how stress and the adrenaline dump affects performance
3. Pain management
4. Mindset

If you're under the impression that you're studying to survive violence but these four elements are not part of your curriculum, you need to quit now and find a system that does teach them.

Understand human nature

To have a better understanding of how to act or react during the pre-physical altercation, you have to become a student of human nature. Recognition of behavioral patterns is paramount. For example, can you recognize Alphas and Betas in a gang situation? An Alpha is the group leader, the decision-maker of the bunch; the rest are Betas, followers, sheep. By the way, generally the more members in a gang the more cowardly each individual is likely to be.

The ability to manipulate human behavior is more important than your ability to punch or kick. Every time you interact with all kinds of people, you get an opportunity to manipulate human behavior. It begins with understanding that 60 percent of communication is body language, 30 percent is tone of voice, and only 10 percent is based on the actual words used to convey the message. If you're a good student of human nature, you know how humans behave in various conditions and situations. You need to have an uncanny sense of observation; you don't need six years of training to become "brutally efficient." Your mind and keen sense of awareness are two things that are going to do it for you.

On being aware

I call this drill, "Noise reaction awareness," one that will enhance your alertness and awareness to your surroundings. Recognize immediately and assess every abrupt noise you hear, i.e., a truck honking, a car screeching, a dog barking. Give the sound a name. Doing this type of exercise randomly a few times a day will exponentially increase your perception time and decrease your reaction time.

Being oblivious to your surroundings or to the body language of your opponent could lead to disaster. For example, there are always pre-contact indicators prior to someone striking:

• heavy or shallow breathing
• looking around subtly
• shifting of weight
• shifting of range (i.e., stepping back or stepping closer)
• tightness of facial features and facial muscles
• grinding of the teeth
• elevation of voice
• stiffness of a limb
• removing of their shirt or jacket
• dropping their bag.

Being familiar with these pre-contact indicators will greatly reduce your chance of being preempted or sucker punched.

Cheating is impossible when there are no rules. An intelligent warrior will attempt to verbally defuse and de-escalate a potentially violent confrontation. He will physically engage only if he has loaded the dice in his favor using all of his psychological tools, everything from simple body language to verbal initiators.

Victim behavior attracts predatory attention; any 10-year-old child watching the *Discovery Channel* knows this. How do you eliminate victim behavior? By being proactive. Knowing how a predator thinks and acts is imperative. You have to look at it from a 3-dimensional perspective. The more you know about your enemy, the easier it is to defeat him. Study, research, and learn to think like a criminal: Where would you attack if you were a sociopath? Acting, bluffing, or role-playing are all strategies to enhance your tactical edge.

Physical conditioning

Where does physical fitness fit into all of this? Bruce Lee said that you can know all the techniques in the world but if you're not physically fit they become useless to you.

Able to keep fighting

Strength (meaning in this case endurance, muscular and emotional) is like a bullet in a gun: If you have lots, you're able to pull the trigger more than if you have only a little. The better conditioned you are the more chances you have of applying plan B when plan A fails, and applying plan C when plan B fizzles. If you're poorly conditioned... well, you're up the proverbial creek when plan A fails.

Imagine this scene: You just finished dropping one opponent when suddenly two of his buddies appear. You run and they chase you for five minutes before they finally corner you. You're exhausted from your first fight, the five-minute run, and the emotional inertia of the situation. Now you have to face two attackers who might be armed. If your fitness level is sub-par, you likely will not leave this situation intact.

Train for it

Pushing yourself physically beyond what you thought you were capable of doing will not only toughen you physically but mentally and emotionally as well. If you cannot go beyond 50 sit-ups, 100 push-ups, or 5 rounds of hard sparring, what on Earth makes you think you will survive a real fight? I'm not talking about your weekly wrestling match with your brother or the average punk who gave you the finger from the car ahead of you. I'm talking about the crack head in the alley with a knife at your throat.

The harder your training sessions, the stronger you become spiritually. You never know what you can do until you've gone beyond what you believed were your limitations. Every time you get lazy or feel fatigued during your workout that is when you push yourself to do more than you think you're capable. Put this on the wall in your training area:

If you have enough energy to whine and complain, you have enough energy to keep on pushing

Commitment

Self-doubt, hesitation and uncertainty will get you killed. Ed Parker said it best: "He who hesitates, meditates horizontally." Commitment to your cause is imperative; you must not "try" to do your best. *Trying* implies possibility of failure, a possibility of being maimed or killed. In *Star Wars: Return of the Jedi*, Yoda said, "*Do*, don't try." When training, you should never stop to redo a drill when you screw up a move; doing this will cause you to short circuit during a real fight. Instead, pick up from wherever you screwed up and continue.

There is a difference between fighting and combat. This is semantics, true enough, but as Dan Millman said, "The conventions of language reveal the ways in which we see the world." To give you an example, when you walk into a traditional dojo or kwoon and ask a student why he is training there, the most common and probable answer is, "To get my black belt." When you enter a school that teaches HTHC, hand-to-hand combat, and ask the same question, you get, "To save my ass in case I get into a scrap."

Killing an individual, even in self-defense, is not something I condone. Getting out of a situation without killing your opponent but knowing that you could have is power. Instead, you can hurt, injure or cripple him to buy you enough time to get away. Besides, more often than not your opponent will not be ready for combat in the spiritual sense; most people don't have the heart for it.

It's said that the only way out of hell is straight through it. Likewise with combat. You know you will get hurt and possibly die, so you have to blast straight through it without hesitation to hurt them more before they hurt you. Avoid killing at all costs.

Self-dense vs. martial arts

There are currently no governing bodies in the martial arts or self-defense field. This makes it frustrating, since anyone who has enough money to rent an empty space, buy a gi, put on a black belt, and hang a few certificates on his wall can claim to teach martial arts. Mistakenly linked with martial arts is the term "self-defense." This is where social responsibility comes in. Most, unfortunately, have none.

Self-defense and martial arts are two completely different animals. Martial arts are divided into various categories: full-contact sports, semi-contact sports, submission sports, and traditional martial arts that do not compete. Not one of these can be labeled self-defense, although most often they all are. It's not to say that a small or large percentage of these styles or systems cannot effectively be used for self-defense, they most certainly can. However, the social irresponsibility lies with the instructor who tags that term on his style or system without proper research. Most believe that their entire style or system is functional as a means of personal protection.

Personal protection or fighting is a complete system of its own. To study a portion of it through styles or systems that are incomplete will leave the individual incomplete. This can lead to disaster.

If a system or style does not holistically address the physical arsenal as well as the psychological and emotional elements of fear, pain, and stress management strategies, then that system or 'style' is only teaching partial preparation and is therefore limiting your survivability. If it doesn't realistically use role playing scenarios and replications, then it's incomplete. If it's labeled as a "style" then it's incomplete.

Totality of combat is achieved when:

- You have fully comprehended the physical applications of each fighting range.

- You have learned how to mesh them when necessary.

- You're fully capable of psychologically manipulating human behavior to your advantage.

- You have control of your emotions and never overreact.

- You can fight in all ranges under all conditions regardless of environment.

- You're in good physical condition.

Once you have achieved a level of proficiency in all of the above bullets, you can go on to expand your knowledge of combatives by further exploring the ranges of combat without developing any kind of preference for any tool, range, or technique. To build a house (to survive a fight) you need hammers, saws, and screwdrivers (strikes, locks, parries, and blocks). You need to know how to use your tools and have a plan (strategy) so the house doesn't crumble a month later. Now, it's pointless to learn how to use a car jack when your objective is to build a house. Likewise, it's pointless to learn a flying armbar when you want to learn how to defend yourself.

Important point: For the sake of survival, don't practice or train in something you will never use.

How you train is how you fight

What you do in the training hall is what you will do in real life; it's called muscle memory. Martial artists who claim, "Well, I know what I would do in a real fight" had better seriously reevaluate that statement. When you train in something long enough it becomes innate. We have had countless students from various martial arts styles train with us and all had developed bad habits - dropping their hands, being too stiff and rigid, or being to linear - that took months to undo. It's not their fault, but the fault of muscle memory; they have done it a certain way for so long that it has become a part of them. Practice does not make perfect, but *proper* practice makes as close to perfect as you will ever get since perfection doesn't exist.

I hope that these concepts and attributes will guide you to a better understanding of hand-to-hand combat. If you have questions or comments please feel free to contact me.

---

*R*ichard Dimitri is considered one of the world's leading authorities on personal protection and hand-to-hand combat. Although still considered very "underground," his programs and drills have been integrated by martial artists, law enforcement, and civilians the world over. His research and martial arts training is backed by experience in which he applied his physical and psychological skills while working as an undercover security guard, a bouncer and bodyguard for high-profile clients for over a decade.

In 1994, Mr. Dimitri opened his educational institution where he and his team teach Senshido's principles and concepts. He had the pleasure of teaching the prestigious SAS, US Marines, Canadian Armed Forces, France's Marine Infantry, LEOs, RCMP officers, Pinkerton Security, VIP Investigations, Tandem Montreal, McGill University's Walksafe department, and bouncers and doormen from several Montreal clubs.

Mr. Dimitri has been featured in several films, magazines, television and radio shows the world over, and he has authored what is considered to be by many experts one of the best books ever written on personal protection, In *Total Defense of the Self*, an international best seller. He also produced over 30 Instructional DVDs considered the most comprehensive and educational self-defense tapes on the market today.

Mr. Dimitri developed the close-quarter conceptual tool known as The Shredder™. It has been referred to as "the missing link in martial arts/self defense" and has been adopted by law enforcement agencies, correctional institutions, military personnel, and martial artists world wide.

People travel yearly from Brazil, Greenland, Finland, Scotland, Germany, Italy, Middle East, Venezuela, UK, Puerto Rico, and the United States to train with Mr. Dimitri. He continues his research and his methods continue to evolve. Contact Mr. Dimitri at www.Senshido.com, at RDimitri@Senshido.com or call 514-979-5621.

Many thanks to Adam Cooper and Julie Mandino for posing with me, and to my excellent photographer, Anthony Lukban.

4 Quick and Effective Sanshou Combinations

An Interview with Wim Demeere
Conducted by Loren W. Christensnen

Loren W. Chistensen (LWC) What do people generally think of when they hear the name, sanshou?

Wim Demeere (WD): Most people don't really know the art under that name. They have usually heard of kung fu, sometimes wushu, but sanshou rarely rings a bell. Though in the last couple of years, sports Sanshou has gained popularity via tournaments and pro-fights that have aired on national television.

In Asia, the name is better known. But even there you can find some confusion when people use sanshou to refer to one specific category (either military, civilian or sports) and feel the other two aren't part of that term. So it does get confusing at times, which is probably one of the biggest hurdles the art has to take before getting better known.

LWC: What is sanshou?

WD: A rough translation of the word sanshou from Chinese would be "free fighting." This could mean many things but in this context, an appropriate definition would be: "Using the fighting applications of Chinese martial arts for self-defense or combat." All martial arts consist of forms, drills, conditioning, and several other aspects, to include the fighting applications. The last one is what sanshou is all about.

Sanshou is usually divided into three categories:

Military Sanshou:

This is the hand-to-hand combat curriculum of the Chinese army; no-nonsense, close-combat fighting for soldiers.

Civilian Sanshou:

On the one hand, this comprises a watered down version of the military techniques since it was developed as a system to give the average civilian effective techniques to defend themselves. There were many changes to the curriculum; for example, a civilian typically has no need for sentry removal techniques.

On the other hand, this category contains the fighting techniques of all the Chinese martial arts as well. From *wing chun* to *hung gar* to *ba ji quan* and all the other hundreds of Chinese styles. Sanshou contains an amazing amount of different flavors of combat material present.

Sports Sanshou:

You can view this as the Chinese version of kickboxing, sometimes called sanda. It's a full-contact sport using punches, knees, kicking, throwing, and stand-up grappling. Sports sanshou has two particularities.

First, there is a focus on putting the opponent on the floor without following him. You lose points if you go to the ground with the other guy. Second, you fight on a raised stage called a "lei tai." This is similar to a boxing ring but without the ropes. If you're forced off the stage two times, you lose the round.

I teach both sports sanshou and combat sanshou, a hybrid style combining techniques from the traditional Chinese arts and sports sanshou.

LWC: How is sanshou similar to karate, taekwondo, kung fu and other kick/punch arts?

WD: It's similar in that some of the techniques of sanshou are found in other arts as well – and vice versa. If something works in combat, chances are it will work just as well in China as it will in Japan, Korea, or any other part in the world. This is valid for striking techniques (using arms and legs), throws, takedowns, and joint locks. There will be similarities but also differences.

For instance, some punches in sanshou are very similar to Western boxing. This came about through the influence Western techniques had on sports sanshou. You now see fighters who have a typical Western style in their punches, more of a Chinese style, or a hybrid that mixes influences from both sides. You can see such similarities and differences across the board of the techniques in sanshou.

However, there are also numerous differences, not as much in techniques per se but more in the way they are expressed. For instance, compared to traditional shotokan karate, sanshou looks a lot more fluid and circular. Compared to taekwondo it has many more arm techniques and throws. Sanshou definitely has a unique flavor to it.

Cycling strikes

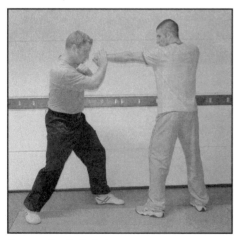

Parry the left jab.

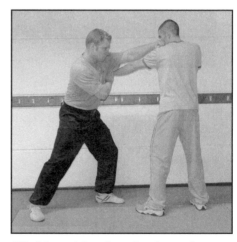

Hit him with a fast, horizontal hammer fist

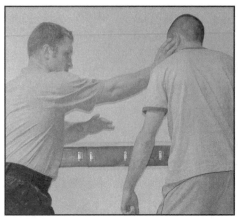

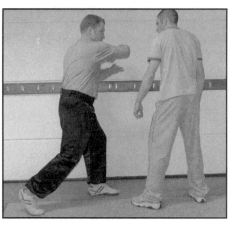

Follow up with a right circular claw to the face. Rip your fingers across as you dig in with them.

Pull the arm completely through so it is poised to strike again.

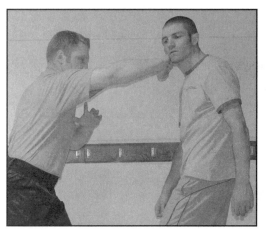

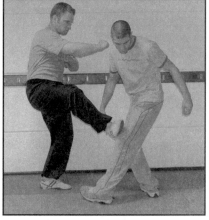

Return on the same angle with a right hammer fist.

Finish with a right stomp kick to the knee.

LWC: Could an observer watch a sanshou practitioner train or fight for, say, three minutes and know that the person is a sanshou practitioner. Is the "unique flavor" you mentioned *that* unique?

WD: It is certainly possible but the observer would have to possess some in-depth knowledge of the art to spot the uniqueness since the signs can be subtle. It might even look like the fighter makes what would be beginner's mistakes in another art. For instance, some fighters like to keep the lead hand very low, like boxers did in the late 19th century. The lead hand then circles a bit and lures the opponent into closing the gap and punching at the face, which seems wide open. As soon as he does so, the sanshou fighter will use that hand for a takedown or throw as he ducks the punch. Nowadays, it's rare to see boxers use such a high-low guard; they figure a guy who does that is an easy target.

 Another subtlety is how a sanshou fighter bends through the knees a little bit more than most other arts. He tries to lower his center of gravity to avoid a counter-throw or sweep as he punches. He also avoids standing on the ball of the foot in most kicking techniques. Where many styles prefer to raise the heel in a roundhouse kick, sanshou doesn't. This slows the kick down a little but you get a lot of stability in return. Many other smaller and larger aspects give that unique flavor when you see them combined together.

LWC: How is it similar to jujitsu?

WD: Many locks in sanshou attack the joints and bone structure of the arms, legs, spine and neck. Joint work is called *chin na* in Chinese arts and is usually a clearly distinguished part of the curriculum. These either control the opponent or break the targeted joint. Depending on the situation, you can go for either one of these options, though in combat sanshou you would rarely go for a controlling lock.

Elbow-locking throw

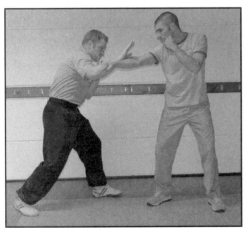

Deflect the attacker's right jab as you step to your left.

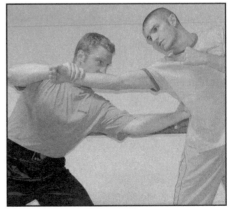

Grab his wrist and fire a right punch to his body.

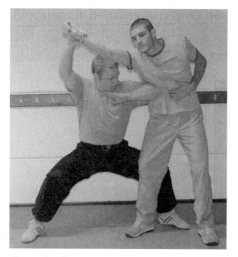 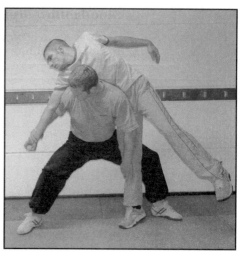

Scoot in for a reverse elbow as you pull his arm upward.

Load him on your upper back or shoulders by hyper extending his elbow on your upper arm and grab his leg with your other hand. Throw him in any direction you desire.

LWC: What is the percentage of kicking/punching to grappling?

WD: It's about 50/50. A good sanshou fighter is comfortable fighting in all ranges. Typically, he prefers to use his legs when at long range, arm techniques in medium range and grappling at close range. But this is more a guideline than a fixed rule.

There are many examples in which you do the opposite: Stomping kicks from medium range, clawing techniques while grappling, and many more. You practice striking and grappling techniques at a specific range first, the distance at which they are the easiest to learn and master. Once you're familiar with them, the goal is to learn all the other distances at which you can apply a specific technique. No matter where you find yourself in relation to your opponent, you should have more than enough options available to you.

Close-range striking to takedown

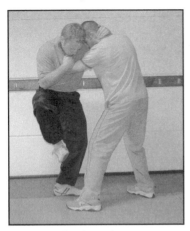

From a clinch, raise your right foot..."

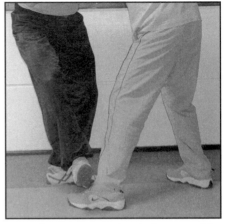

...and stomp your heel down on his foot or ankle."

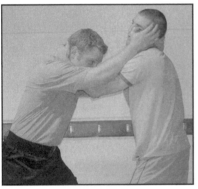

Put your right leg back for stability and shove his face back by thumbing him in the eye.

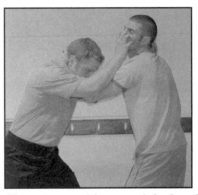

Claw down with your right hand.

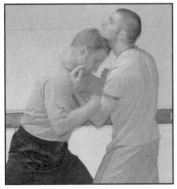

Follow with an upward head butt to his chin.

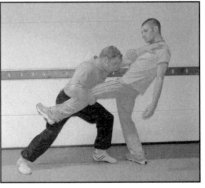

Grab his lead leg and lift it as you shove him back off balance.

LWC: How open is sanshou to accepting techniques from other styles?

WD: This depends on the mindset of both the practitioner and his teacher. Generally, the Chinese have always been hesitant to allow outside influences to their arts, although this seems to be changing ever so slowly. Personally, I think it's a matter of understanding the art you learn before mixing other influences in it. If it makes sense to add something, by all means, you should go for it. But if it isn't compatible then why would you? Then we come back to the original premise; do you have enough knowledge of the art itself to alter its curriculum? Everyone has to answer this for himsef.

LWC: What is your approach to sanshou? Sport? Street? A mix of the two?

WD: The system I teach, combat sanshou, is a mixture of both. The parts from sports Sanshou are the full-contact sparring and specific techniques such as good boxing skills, powerful kicking techniques and practical throwing/grappling skills. The street orientation is when I add those vicious techniques from traditional arts: clawing, joint breaking, eye gouging and numerous other techniques that would get you banned for life from a competitive arena.

The goal is to combine the best of both worlds: you become accustomed to adrenal stress by fighting full-power (under controlled circumstances) but you also learn skills that go way beyond the context of a sports tournament, skills that prepare you for the street.

LWC: What are sanshou's limitations for the street?

WD: A key aspect is the legal and moral responsibility. Some of the techniques are extremely brutal. Instead of merely knocking down your opponent, you punish him with crippling techniques so he can't get up anymore. These are taught in a sub-section called "finishing moves." As the name implies, they are meant to end the fight right then by causing excessive injuries.

The limitation is that you can't just break somebody's elbows and shoulders because he gave you a look you don't like. You have to be legally justified to do such a technique. If you are not, you will probably spend years or even the rest of your life behind bars.

In our modern society we tend to forget that traditional arts come from a different era. A few hundred years ago China was a different place from today. If you didn't have the skills to defend your town and family from murdering and pillaging bandits, you simply died. You couldn't dial 911 and wait for help to arrive. In that context, extremely violent techniques make perfect sense. They are not meant for the ring, or for a situation in which you can choose less brutal options. You only use them when you have no other choice left but to go to an extreme to survive a violent attack.

The moral responsibility is that you have to learn when you can and when you can't use such techniques. Distinguishing between these situations is difficult as you never know how a street confrontation will turn out. In a majority of street altercations, there is no need for extremes though. But if you have to go there, you'll be prepared.

LWC: Do you see this ever changing? Right now it doesn't seem that sanshou would be good for law enforcement or anyone just wanting to learn how to control someone, as opposed to destroying their limbs with finishing moves.

WD: It isn't that you have to use a brutal move to finish a fight. As I said before, more often than not, you don't need to go that far. But combat sanshou specifically prepares you for the eventuality. If your goal is to control an attacker or you don't want to hurt him, you shouldn't focus on the finishing moves. That is why sanshou fighters love to put opponents on the floor. The throw or sweep can be enough to knock the wind out of somebody, especially if he falls on a hard surface. If it doesn't, you're in an ideal position for additional techniques should he want to resume the fight. But the choice is yours; you can be merciful or you can be harsh, depending on how the opponent reacts.

Another option is to practice the joint locks, chin na, to a larger degree. Chin na has a wide variety of techniques and drills that teach you all the joint locks you might possibly need to control an aggressor. Once again the choice is yours to control or break the joint, depending on the actions of your opponent.

LWC: What are sanshou's weaknesses?

WD: Sanshou is well rounded when it comes to striking and stand-up grappling, but compared to systems like Greco-Roman wrestling or shoot fighting, the ground grappling isn't as well developed. Those other systems have a far more complex and diversified range of joint locks and choke holds on the ground than sanshou.

Stay on your feet

In sanshou, you never go to the ground if you can prevent it. When you come into clinching or grappling range, you always do so with the goal of staying in an upright position with both feet firmly planted on the floor. This is true for both a self-defense situation in the street and in full-contact competitions. You want the other guy to eat dirt but without dirtying your clothes by rolling on the ground with him.

The reason is simple: Chinese arts tend to think of a downed opponent as a dead man. Referring back to previous centuries again, if you fell to the floor during a fight, you were stomped or the attacker ran you through with a sword or spear. It's rather difficult to defend against a 25-inch-long blade being stuck in your guts when you're lying down. That's why Chinese fighters prefer to put the opponent on the floor without following him there. They prefer a stand up position and finish the guy off from there.

There are some exceptions to this. Certain Chinese styles have techniques for fighting from the ground, but they don't have the depth and breadth of those other grappling systems that focus heavily on groundwork.

LWC: What are sanshou's strengths?

WD: Sanshou has two strong points that are interwoven: downing the opponent and stability. The overall goal, the main strategy, is to put the other guy on the floor – hard - without going there yourself. All the techniques are set-ups for that goal; everything you do leads to breaking his balance and dumping him on the ground. This is a highly successful strategy both in the ring and on the street.

The key ingredient for this formula is stability. If you aren't in balance, it's hard to destabilize your opponent and avoid falling to the ground yourself. In sport sanshou you even lose points when you fall on top of your opponent during a throw, or if you take too long to get back on your feet. These things can get you inured or worse in the streets. Sanshou spends tons of training time on the ability to stay in balance under pressure.

Recover from failed takedown

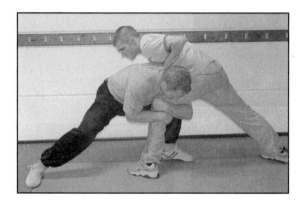

The opponent blocks your takedown by taking a step back and shoving you down.

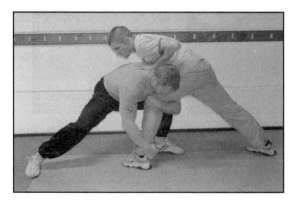

Remain stationary and grab his lead ankle with your right hand.

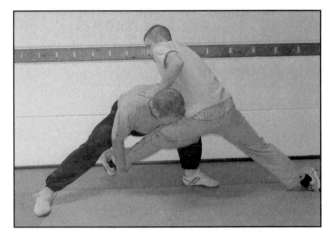

Apply leverage by pulling at his lead ankle as you shove your lead shoulder into his hips.

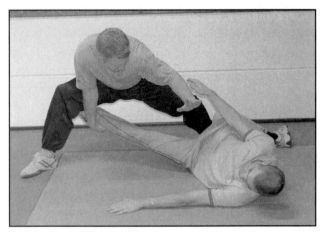

Pull his foot against your upper leg to control it as you guard against any incoming attacks.

LWC: Are there kicks?

WD: There are numerous kicking techniques such as the well-known front, side and roundhouse kicks. But also stomping, knee strikes, shin kicks and scoop kicks. The strategy is limited to certain specific situations:

Long range:

Your legs are longer than your arms so it makes sense to exploit this reach advantage.

Medium and close range:

This isn't sanshou's preferred kicking range for power. In that distance we use our legs to surprise our opponent or complement arm techniques; for instance, when both your hands are busy controlling the other guy, you can still kick or knee him.

The crucial skill as far as kicking goes is retracting the leg as fast as you shoot it out. If you're sloppy and the retraction is slow, he will catch your leg or hit you when you're still balancing on one leg. This is a standard defense in sanshou against kicking techniques and we assume that the other guy will try to do that to us when we use our legs. With that in mind, the retraction phase becomes almost more important as actually kicking the other guy.

LWC: Can you train sanshou solo?

WD: You most certainly can. Solo practice is an integral and important part of the curriculum. You do it to ingrain techniques so they become natural but you also do it to keep getting better and better at the thousands of little details that make the difference between a *good* and a *great* technique.

I start every single workout with some sort of solo training. It might be shadow boxing or repeating a single technique a hundred times. There is always something to work on. In every session, I typically discover a small tweak that makes the technique more effective or I spot an error I didn't realize had crept into my punch or kick.

Solo training is probably the truest test of character for the martial artist. There is no blaming your partner when you mess up or no making excuses that the opponent is too strong; it's all about overcoming the limitations you perceive in your own mind, spirit and body.

---

*W*im Demeere began training in the martial arts at the age of 14, studying the grappling arts of judo and jujitsu for several years before turning to the kick/punch arts of traditional kung fu and its full-contact competitions. He studied a traditional Chinese style called hung chia pai, which is renowned for its ruthless training methods and emphasis on body conditioning. It also gave him a strong foundation in traditional Chinese free-fighting and self defense techniques called sanshou. This style was a steppingstone to research the sanshou systems of many different Chinese arts.

Over the years, Wim has studied a broad range of other fighting styles, including muay Thai, kali, pentjak silat and shootfighting. Since the late 1990s, he has been studying combat tai chi chuan.

Wim Demeere's competitive years saw him win four national titles and a bronze medal at the 1995 World Wushu Championships. In 2001, he became the national coach of the Belgian Wushu fighting team.

A full-time personal trainer in his native country of Belgium, Mr. Demeere instructs both business executives and athletes in nutrition, strength and endurance, and a variety of martial arts styles. He has managed a corporate wellness center and regularly gives lectures and workshops in the corporate world.

As an author, Mr. Demeere has co-authored two books with Loren W. Christensen: *The Fighter's Body: An Owner's Manual* and *Timing in the Fighting Arts: Your Guide to Winning in the Ring and in the Streets.*

You can contact Mr. Demeere through his website The Grinding Shop at www. grindingshop.com

Thanks to Roan Van Boeckel for posing as the opponent and to Dirk Crokaert for his hard work behind the camera.

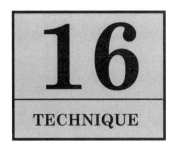

8 Ways to Stomp

By Loren W. Christensen

Admittedly, the word "stomp" has a negative connotation. Stomping on a helpless victim is something bullies, gangbangers, and prisoners do. It's what a mob does, people who get their courage by virtue of their numbers. While all these are true, there are also times when stomps are a viable part of self-defense. In fact, there are times when it's the very technique that will save your day.

Now, there isn't anything terribly complicated about stomping although there is a bit of a knack to it. With proper body mechanics, you can stomp with tremendous force.

The mechanics

How not to stomp

Often, fighters stomp by thrusting their foot down onto a target while lifting their upper bodies. Their foot goes down and their upper body goes up. This divides their energy. Part of it is going one way and part of is going the other.

Your energy divides when you take someone to the ground and then jerk his

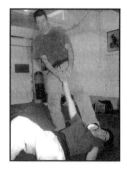

arm upward as you stomp down on him. Your foot goes down and your upper body goes up. Energy divided. Additionally, if you have ever executed this move and missed, you know why the cry "Agghh! I've hyperextended my knee" was invented.

Know why you're stomping

As mentioned throughout this book, there always needs to be justification for you to use force, especially to stomp someone. The word "stomp" connotes that the stomper is standing and the stompee is on the ground. The police, district attorney, and a jury are going to wonder why, since you were standing, you didn't run away when the assailant fell or was thrown to the ground.

Stomping because you were mad at the guy isn't going to cut it with the authorities. You need to be able to articulate in what way the threat was still a danger to you as he lay on the ground. For example:

• He had a gun in his hand.

• He had a knife in his hand and he was starting to get up.

• Before the attacker fell, he was clearly dominating you. The fall didn't hurt him and he was getting back up again.

• He uttered threats that he was going to hurt or kill you as he tried to get up.

• You had knocked him to the ground previously and he had gotten up every time. This time he had retrieved a weapon from a pocket

How to stomping from the ground to use as a weapon.

I began rethinking the stomp after hearing J. Kelly McCann, a real-world martial arts instructor, author, and CNN commentator discuss the very issue I just described in "How not to stomp." McCann's remedy isn't as pretty looking as the way you shouldn't do it but it does deliver tremendous impact.

One-legged stomp

I like this method best because I feel I have good balance and control of my body when landing on something, like an arm or leg.

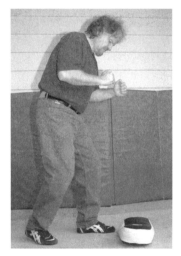

Stand with your left leg forward.

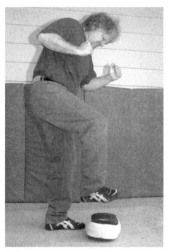

Move your right foot past your left as you crouch a little.

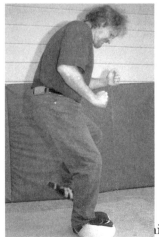

Lift your left foot as your right foot stomps downward. Simultaneous with the stomp, crouch a little more to facilitate dropping your weight and energy into the target. Try bending your arms and clenching your fists as pictured to make your body heavy. Stomp again if needed or back quickly out of range.

ight help your coordination to think of lifting your

non-stomping leg the same way you think of retracting your hand when you punch. No, it's not dividing your force, but rather facilitating the speed of your stomp.

No energy bleed

Palm-heel someone in the face while they are standing and their head snaps back and they either fall down or stagger back a few steps. I have no clue what the percentage breakdown would be, but part of the impact's energy goes into the recipient's head and the other goes out into the air, out into the empty space behind the person. Let's call that energy bleed.

However, palm-heel that head when it's braced by a wall and all of the impact energy, or virtually all of it, goes into the head. There is no energy bleed out into the air behind the target.

The same thing happens when you stomp a target supported by the floor. The entire impact goes into the arm, ankle, head or whatever you slam.

That makes your stomp really, really hurt.

Two-legged stomp

Remember that scene in *Enter the Dragon* when Bruce Lee leaped into the air and then came down onto his opponent in a two-legged stomp? Do you remember the slow motion contorted face that Bruce made and that panther-like scream? Well, those things are optional when doing a two-legged stomp.

What isn't optional is that you strive to deliver as much impact as you're able.

Here is a good way to do it.

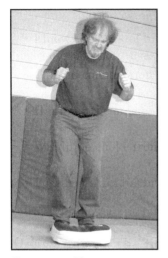

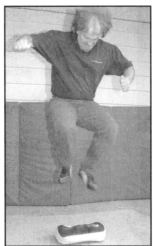

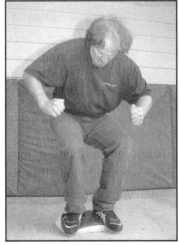

Set yourself.

Jump. You don't have to go this high but it's good practice.

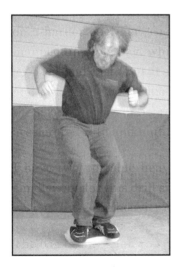

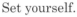

Land in a slight crouch with arms bent and hands fisted.

As with the one-legged stomp, the slight crouch and the tense upper body increases the impact. But don't let that impact get trapped in your upper half. Mentally force your energy down through your legs and into the target. This helps you deliver greater force and helps your stability when landing on a round target, such as an arm or thigh.

Important point: Whether you stomped with one or both feet, hit again if it's needed, lock-up the person with a control hold, or scoot quickly out of range. He might have tolerated your technique and now he is really mad because you left a foot print on his clothes. If you're not executing a follow-up move, get out of range. Even better, run.

Target selection

This isn't rocket science; it's quite easy to figure out what body part would hurt when someone stomps on it with prejudice. But keep in mind that because there is a floor, sidewalk, or street underneath the target, the entire stomp is absorbed into the body part. So, just about any place you stomp is going to hurt. Still, some targets are especially vulnerable to pain and damage when supported by something underneath them.

When opponent is lying face up

- Face
- Mouth
- Fingers
- Biceps
- Groin
- Shin
- Side of foot
- Nose
- Neck chest
- Inside elbow
- Stomach
- Upper thigh
- Top of ankle

When opponent is lying face down

- Back of head
- Fingers
- Triceps
- Coccyx bone
- Calf
- Ankle
- Back of neck
- Elbow
- Kidneys
- Back of thigh
- Achilles tendon
- Toes

Also, keep in mind that a heavily muscled body part, a body part covered with pounds of blubber, or one covered with a heavy winter coat, will likely be more tolerant of impact. A well-padded upper arm or thigh might require two or three stomps before the attacker stops trying to get up, or calls out, "I give up." Or, you might stomp it once because it's the only target open at that precise moment, and then when others open up as a result of his reaction, you can deliver a second stomp to a less padded body part.

Let's look at five simple scenarios in which you can deliver a stomp to hopefully end a confrontation.

To take out an attacker's support base:

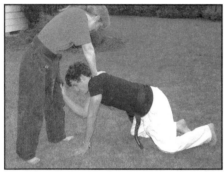

You have dumped the attacker onto the ground, but he grabs your leg when you start to escape.

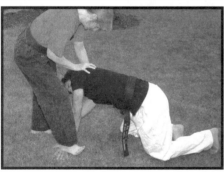

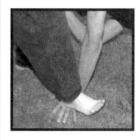

Stomp the fingers of his support hand

To injure an attacker's means to pursue:

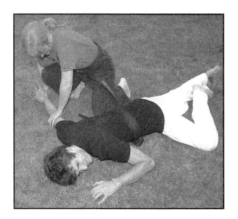

You have taken the attacker down twice during the fight, but he keeps getting up and coming after you. Again you have taken him down onto his belly.

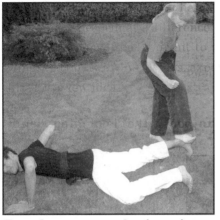

Stomp his Achilles' tendon as you flee.

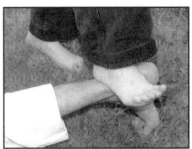

To reduce an attacker's resistance

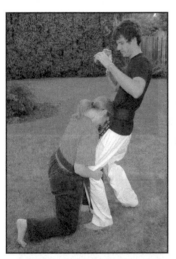

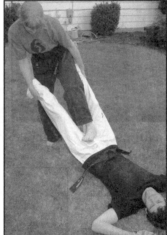

You shoot in for a double knee yank. (left)

The instant he lands, stomp the closest target, the groin. (right)

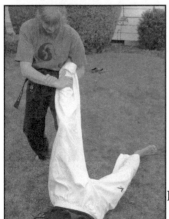

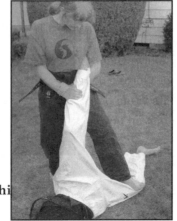

Apply a figure-4 calf lock... (left)

...and stomp his other thigh, or his groin again to take any residual fight out of him. (right)

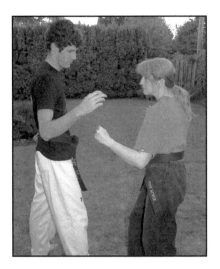 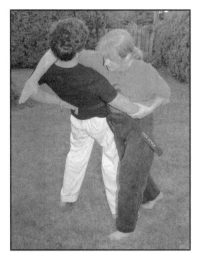

The instant the attacker moves his arm behind him to retrieve a weapon, execute a bent-arm clothesline takedown.

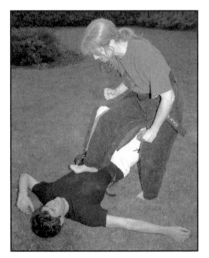 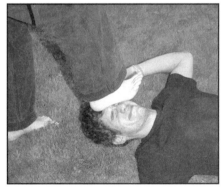

... and then stomp his head to slow his pursuit.

The instant he lands, stomp the closest target...

People are funny. You smash a deserving person in the face and onlookers say, "Good for you. The jerk deserved it." But knock the "jerk" down onto the floor and stomp that same face, some people are turned off. "Yeah," they say, "the guy was a creep and he shouldn't have hit you with a bottle, but he didn't deserve to be stomped." It's all about perception and connotation. As mentioned at the beginning of this chapter, some people view stomping as something that bullies do. Sophisticated people don't stomp.

It's similar to the days of the Old West where an ethical cowboy rancher would never shoot another guy in the back, no matter how despicable the man. Even when I was a kid watching westerns, I never understood that rational. Why not shoot him? The bad guy had a gun in his hand. He just shot the sheriff and the parson. Just because he is looking the other way was, in my 12-year-old mind, no reason for the rancher not to plug him. What if the bad guy spun quick as a flash and could shoot accurately? Sure, the town's folks saw the procrastinating rancher as ethical, but now he would be dead ethical.

My point here is that among some people there is a negative connotation attached to stomping. If this is an issue with you, think about it. If it's something you just cannot do, then you need to train accordingly. You need to ask: What am I going to do when I'm standing, the assailant is on the floor at my feet, and the situation dictates that I do something to prevent his further aggression? What can I do when I'm cornered, he is still armed, or he is trying to pull me down onto him? What are some alternative techniques that stop the threat as efficiently and quickly as do stomps? If you're stuck, you might want to revisit stomps.

---

*L*oren W. Christensen's biography appears in the "About the Author" page at the back of the book.

Many thanks to Lisa Christensen and Alex Larson for demonstrating the techniques. I operated the camera.

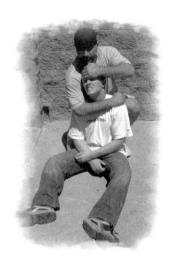

SECTION FOUR
GRAPPLING

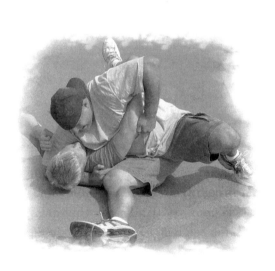

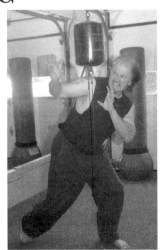

GRAPPLING

20 Ways to Fight in the Clinch

By Mark Mireles

"The clinch." Made popular by professional mixed martial arts (MMA) events such as the UFC and Pride Fighting Championships, these two words have become as common as "punch" and "kick." We have heard the MMAs' commentators and the fighters themselves talk about controlling the clinch, a position that resembles standing wrestling. Terms such as "over-under," "body lock," "pummeling," and "dirty boxing" are all used in conjunction with the words, the clinch.

Is the clinch unique to professional MMA? How important is it to fighting in the real world? Will you see it on the street?

Because of my mixed martial arts training and my experience in street fighting, I firmly believe that the clinch is a natural dynamic of real hand-to-hand combat. If a fight lasts for more than a few minutes, the combatants, both experienced and inexperienced, will inevitably lock onto each other in a clinch. It might not be a technically sound one, but that is a matter or training and understanding. The bottom line is that the position is relevant to street fighting and it's a tactic worthy of study.

Personally I believe much of the clinch fighting we see in MMA is relevant to street fighting. I take the competition aspects of the clinch out of my training and teaching curriculum, and I focus on street situations, tactics and techniques. MMA as a sport is rough and tumble with many cross-over techniques, principles and concepts that relate to the street. Clinch fighting is one of them.

The street fighting clinch, based on MMA training methods, is applicable to hand-to-hand combat, edged weapon defense, firearms retention and disarms. It's broad based when you consider the totality of violent scenarios on the street. This chapter will focus on the basics of this position.

The Greco-Roman model for clinch fighting

In my experience, the clinch is an area not well understood by marital artists. There is little written on the subject and there are only a few instructors who incorporate practical clinch fighting into their curriculum. I'll even go so far as to say that many fighters don't know where the position originated (in the international Olympic styles of wrestling, in case anyone asks).

Of the two forms of international wrestling - Greco-Roman and freestyle - only the Greco-Roman school of wrestling focuses on the clinch, a style that allows holds *only* above the waist. Freestyle wrestling, however, allows leg and upper body attacks, an approach that is visibly a much different form of wrestling than Greco-Roman.

The restriction of holds to those above the waist in the Greco-Roman system has made upper body wrestling extremely technical. Because the clinch is a constant, Greco Roman practitioners are well-practiced at attacking from it, primarily focusing on attacks to the head, shoulders, upper extremities, and the torso. Their arsenal consists of technical throws, drags, body locks, slides, and off balancing techniques.

In the United States, freestyle wrestling is the dominant style with a significantly fewer number of wrestlers practicing Greco-Roman. The clinch position isn't a high probability in freestyle wrestling, so less training is devoted to it.

Which one is better for the street?

Since freestyle wrestling allows attacks above and below the waist and Greco-Roman wrestling allows holds only above the waist, it would seem logical that freestyle would transfer better into real fighting.

But I've observed the contrary to be true, that Greco-Roman wrestling is the superior system that acts as a gateway to the execution of other techniques from other fighting systems.

In real fights, combatants can hit and kick, but while the freestyle stance is good for attacking any part of the body, it's not designed to defend against hand and feet attacks since the sport doesn't allow striking. Greco-Roman wrestling, however, segues fluidly to other combative techniques. The restricted style is more applicable to real fighting. How did I arrive at this conclusion? Let's break it down further.

The real issue is how fighting unfolds and the type of techniques that are used. It's not that freestyle wrestling doesn't have effective offensive attacks, but its low stance stance makes its practitioner highly vulnerable to strikes.

In particular, the freestyle stance leads with the face. In addition, the freestyle wrestler isn't always in close contact with his opponent. So when he darts in for a takedown from a distance, he leads with his face, a deficiency in the style that can be exploited by a fighter with just a little training.

Clinch basics

The clinch is a position of close contact from which you can grapple and execute strikes. It's not a technique, but rather a position that occurs during the dynamics of a fight, usually between two fighters, though it can also occur in multiple attack situations.

Let's begin by reviewing a few basics, something every good martial artist should continually do.

Stance and movement

Let's use the Greco-Roman stance as our model from which we make the street adjustments.

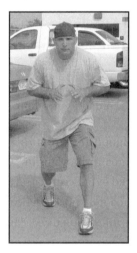

The raw Greco-Roman stance begins with your head up, your back erect, and your shoulders rolled forward to support your neck. Bend your arms at a 90-degree angle and hold them in front of your body. It's important that you keep your elbows tight to your sides. Your thumbs nearly touch in front of your torso.

From an overhead view, note that your arms should form a "V." When you raise your hands to jaw level, the Greco-Roman stance becomes a striker's guard. Your legs are staggered with the forward foot under your hands. Your toes face your adversary.

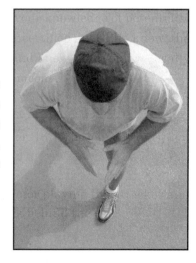

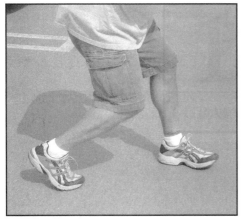

Mobility from the staggered stance comes from flexion in your knees, which is key to maintaining balance. This stance allows you to move forward into your opponent by advancing the front foot two or three inches, trailed by the rear foot.

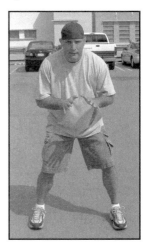

To move laterally. Move your feet to a "square" stance, and then move. Your feet should be wider than your hips. Again, maintain slight flexion in your knees for a balanced stance.

When clinching, you'll be constantly moving your legs from the staggered position to the lateral position to gain advantage and to attack. Keep these points in mind so that both positions feel natural when you move:

- When you switch your legs from staggered to lateral, be sure that your upper body maintains the same position as outlined above.

- Use small shuffling steps when moving laterally.

- Maintain your center of balance at your hips (about two inches below your belly button).

- Never cross your legs when moving and never take large, exaggerated steps.

Attacking the five limbs

A key concept in my clinch methodology is to use upper body wrestling attacks to set up takedowns, throws, and strikes. Let's look at a concept that will help you facilitate the learning curve of clinch work. I call it "attacking limbs," a way of breaking your opponent down into targets for you to attack.

Your opponent has five limbs: two arms, two legs and, what I call the fifth extremity, the head. As you advance in your clinch work, it's helpful to look at your opponent as nothing more than five limbs.

Hand fighting and attacks from the open

The close contact position of the clinch starts with hand fighting, which means for the purpose of clinch work, your ability to seize control of your opponent's wrist and hand. Controlling your opponent's hand is vital in the initial stages of clinch fighting.

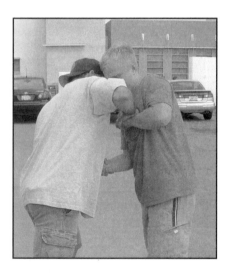
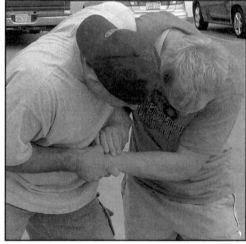

It's important to maintain the wrists or meaty portions of your opponent's hands, no matter from which angle you're grabbing him. Grab him with strong crushing power.

Heavy hands:

This is the beginning of your set-up and the beginning of making life uncomfortable for your opponent.

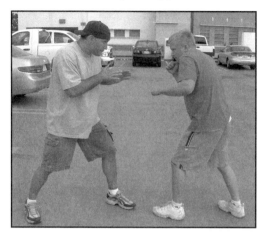

This position is called the "open," a place from which clinch work really begins and where there are many opportunities for attack. Your targets here are the arms and the head of your opponent.

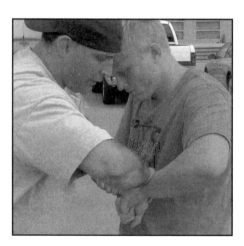
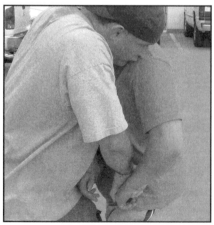

From the open position, grab the top of your opponent's wrists with your palms facing downward. Maximize the strength of this position by pressing down with your hands, a move called "heavy hands." Not only are you pressing them downward but you're placing your body weight onto your opponent's arms and, indirectly, onto his entire body. Heavy hands technique causes the arms of your opponent to straighten, which provides you with two attack options.

The arm drag attack:

The arm drag is the first position of attack from hand fighting.

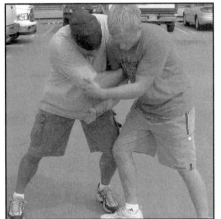

From the heavy hands position, release one wrist and immediately reach deeply into your opponent's opposite armpit. Use your heavy hand on his wrist to feed his arm across the front of your torso. Pull the arm through from the high drag on the armpit while feeding the arm through from the wrist.

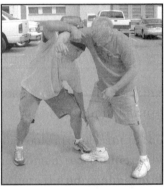

Note the oblique angle created from the arm drag.

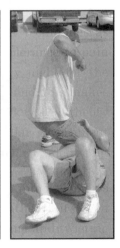

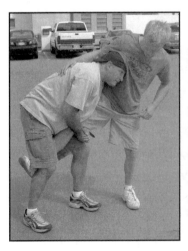
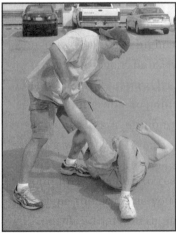
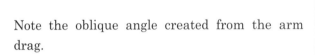

From the oblique angle, you can follow-up with many options, such as dumping him onto his back and pummeling him.

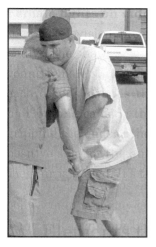 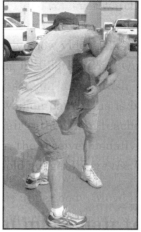 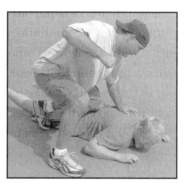

Variation: From the same oblique position, you can take him down onto his belly.

The underhook attack series:

The second attack from heavy hands is the underhook series, a strong position of advantage from which you can execute takedowns and strikes.

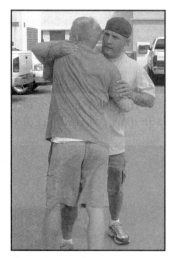 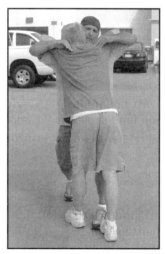

Attack with the single underhook...

... or the double underhook.

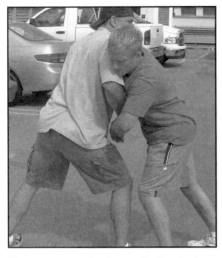 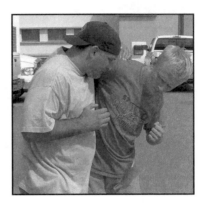

To set up a single underhook from heavy hands, dig your wrist underneath your opponent's shoulder, and hook. In the right photo above, I've opened up my position so you can see the hook better. This action almost resembles an uppercut.

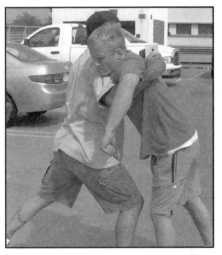

Variation: Secure one side with the double underhook, and then dig with the opposite arm the same way.

Front Headlock attack:

You can use the single underhook to execute a front headlock.

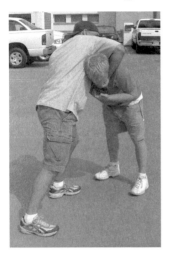

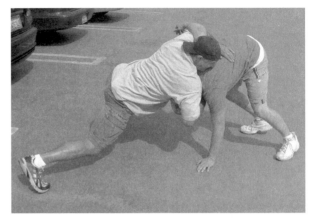

Maintain the underhook as you use your opposite arm to wrap over his head and grab his chin.

Keep weight on your opponent by continuing to sprawl.

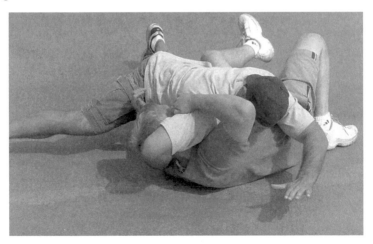

Use the underhook and the chin hold to maneuver your opponent onto his back.

The pinch headlock from the single underhook:

Use this to secure your opponent's head and arm.

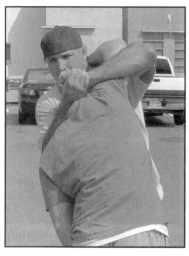

This position creates tremendous pressure on your opponent's shoulder.

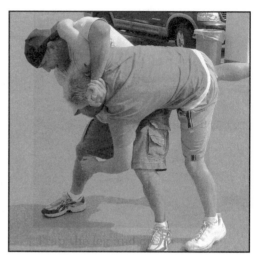

You can twist either way to...

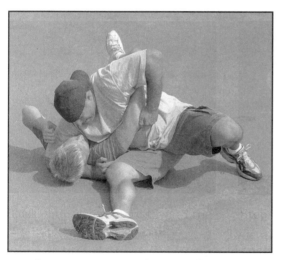

...take your opponent down to the ground.

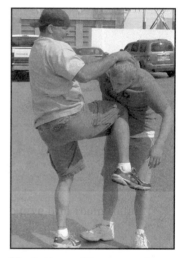

Variations: Short punches and knee strikes are also effective from the single underhook.

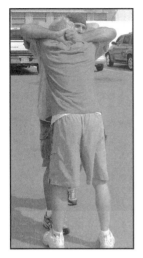

Lock and attack from the double underhook:

Go high. Lock your opponent's elbows high by elevating yours. From here, you can easily execute a throw by twisting your torso. It's the high elbow position that makes the twist so powerful.

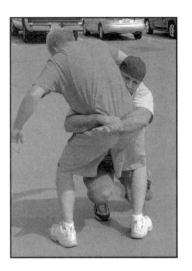

Shoot low. Body-tackle your opponent at waist level to apply the low lock.

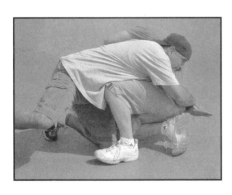

Penetrate into your opponent, a move that resembles a double-leg attack. Note the position of the palms-down lock, a highly effective technique when used in conjunction with the body lock. Drive your hands down while driving forward. Your attacker should fall backwards over his hips.

Important point 1: Never lock your arms in the center of your opponent's back as doing so makes you highly susceptible for your opponent's locking counter throws.

Important point 2: This technique works when there is tremendous downward driving pressure on your opponent's hips as you ram forward with your legs.

Close contact over-under position of the clinch

It's the close contact position of clinch work where martial artists have the most problems. The name "over-under" comes from the position of your arms in the clinch. It's upper body wrestling in its purest form; a position in which you will find yourself in training and in street fighting.

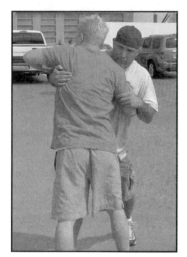

Wrap one of your arms over one of your opponent's arms and slip your other arm under his other one. Your opponent mirrors the same position. Be sure to keep your head up, back erect, knees in slight flexion, and one leg forward.

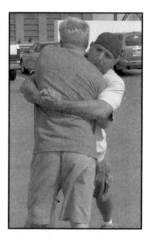

Lock your hands around your opponent's back to tighten the position.

The ability to successfully attack from these positions is what separates the beginner from the veteran clinch fighter. It's one of the more difficult fighting positions to master, as it requires the precise ability to off balance your opponent and throw him.

Attacking from the over-under position

A saying among wrestlers is "The best Greco wrestlers cheat with their legs," which means that although the rules prohibit using the legs, a resourceful wrestler still finds ways to use (cheat) with them. Of course, on the street there are no rules, so you're going to use your legs from the over-under position to execute upper body attacks. From this position, your legs are key to disrupting the balance of your opponent so you can set up successful throws.

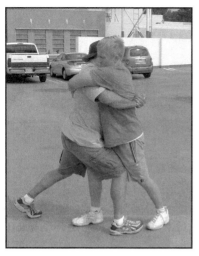

From the over-under position, move your forward leg deep between your opponent's legs. It's doesn't matter which of your legs because you should be well-skilled with an over-under lock with either one in between. Use your lead leg to get a superior position of balance under your opponent's hips. Note the control and deep position. From here, use your leg to off balance your opponent with subtle attacks to his legs. You can also attack his upper body and take him to the ground. Let's break this down with photographs.

The right knee attack

Think of this motion as similar to putting out a cigarette with your foot.

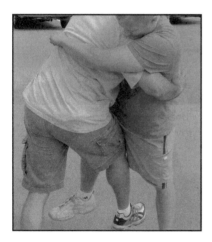

The forward knee attack, or "pop" as it sometimes called, is a quickstep and outer heel twist of your forward foot. This action doesn't have to be an exaggerated motion to work. The twist of the foot pops your attacker's leg up so that he has to balance on one leg.

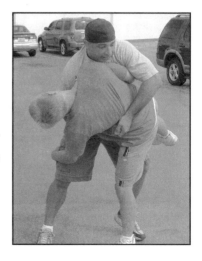

Continue the action in the same direction by twisting your over-under arm position in the same direction.

The left knee attack:

The left knee attack is a more powerful thigh-to-thigh attack and twist.

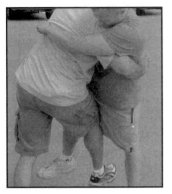

From the over-under position, place your lead, right leg between your opponent's legs. The action of the clinch brings you to a square stance.

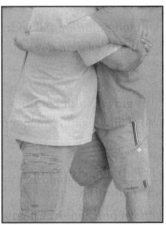

Quickly switch lead legs and attack thigh-to-thigh with your left leg.

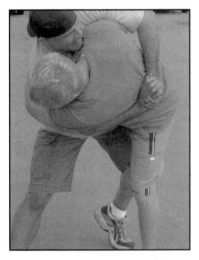

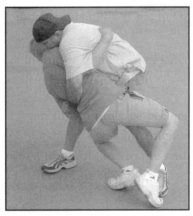

Upon hard thigh-to-thigh contact, pop your hips forward to force your opponent's body to begin a corkscrew motion. Twist your over-under lock in the same direction until he falls on his back.

Important point: Thrust a knee into his torso when you need to soften him prior to the forward knee pop and the rear knee pop.

When all else fails apply the rear suicide scissors

This technique is one of the best ways to take an opponent to the ground quickly. I like to think of it as a last effort attempt because of the large commitment involved. That said, it still has a high probability of success; it just requires a "burn the ships" commitment in your attack. Practice it well.

From the over-under body lock, shoot your forward leg around your opponent's leg on the same side as the arm you have trapped. You have two options:

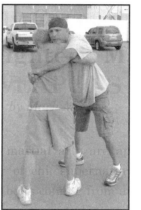 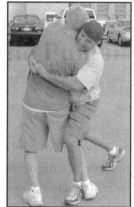

Hook the closest leg...

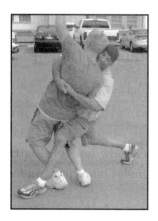 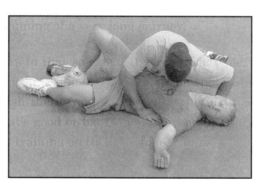

...or hook both legs. When you cut out your opponent's leg(s), he falls onto his back. Once you commit yourself to this action, you have to follow all the way to the ground.

The above positions and attacks are all proven clinch-fighting techniques. While there are numerous other attacks from the clinch, I chose the ones shown here because of their high probability for success in an actual fight. Practice reinforces techniques. Clinch work is no exception. In this final section, I introduce drills and methods to develop your clinch work to a fine precision.

The MMA format for skill building

Clinch fighting is a constant struggle to take control. Let's look at drills that will help you gain proficiency, beginning with a concept I call "pummeling."

Pummeling

"Pummeling" is a term that describes the close-quarter struggle to gain control of your opponent using a series of under-hooks. Unlike the stagnate position depicted in the above photographs, your opponent will attempt to secure under-hooks as you attempt to gain control. It's best to learn pummeling initially in a drill format with light resistance. When you get more conformable with it you can make the drill more intense.

You and your partner start from the open over-under position with your elbows held in close to your body. Alternate the open stance position in a rhythmical rocking motion from side-to-side with light resistance. Take note of the pics to ensure that your stances are correct, in particular, your head, arms, and forward leg. As you warm up, increase tension.

Active pummeling

Active pummeling is a free-form attack and defense using the same pulling action. Go for 5 minutes at 60 to 80 percent effort. Keep the action on your feet; there are no throws or takedowns in this format. The resistance makes you and your partner work hard. When you snag a good hold or position let go and start again. You will quickly get comfortable with this good bridge builder.

3-and-3 drilling

This drill is a skill builder. 3-and-3 means you're going to execute 3 techniques with light resistance, then your training partner executes 3. Repeat the 3-and-

3 exchange and do 25 to 50 reps. Choose any technique you want to work on; let's make it the arm drag. From the clinch, execute 3 arm drags in a row on your cooperative partner and then he immediately executes 3 arm drags.

It's repetition training that builds muscle memory and 3-and-3 is one of the best drills to ingrain a technique. As you learn other clinch attacks, drill them with the 3-and-3 format. It works wonders.

Situational drilling

Often overlooked, situational drilling is nonetheless one of the better training devices that is 100 percent live action. When working on clinches, limit your techniques to only grappling ones. Set the clock for 10 seconds, and then secure a hold on your partner, say, the locked, double underhook. You have 10 seconds to take him down.

Here is the benefit: If you wrestle live for 10 minutes, you might get one or two good under-hooks during that time. While live wrestling has its place, situation drilling can expose you to 30 or more under-hooks in 10 minutes.

Live wrestling

The term "live" means all-out sparring at 100 percent intensity. Start from the over-under body lock and wrestle for a predetermined time limit, though not less than 3 minutes. Wrestle hard and keep attacking.

MMA training for clinch work

In this drill, you simulate the street fighting aspects of the clinch and incorporate all the above drills. You and your training partner don 16-oz boxing gloves and mouthpieces and begin from the over-under position of the clinch. Then go for it. Grapple all-out, but limit your punches to about 50 percent impact, go light with your knee strikes, and refrain from using elbow strikes.

Pad and bag drills

Effective clinch fighting uses inside strikes, which you can perfect on the bags since you can hit them full force. You will want to concentrate your efforts on holding and hitting, which is the art of integrating strikes and standing grappling. Known as "dirty boxing," holding and hitting is an effective method of target softening for street fighting. Here are a few.

- With bag gloves and pads, you can deliver short punches while under-hooking with the opposite hand.

- Use focus mitts and a heavy bag to work your short punching combinations and practice your knee thrusts on larger pads while applying an under-hook.

- Practice short elbow strikes on the heavy bag.

- Practice holding and hitting from as many angles as you can devise.

The clinch is as inevitable in a real fight as skinned knuckles and knees. Many fighters fear it but only because they don't have the knowledge of what all can be done from it. Use the techniques in this chapter as a starting point to understanding the potential you have for dominance in a clinch. Then train and train some more until you own it.

Mark **Mireles** began his study of martial arts over 30 years ago. He has trained in judo, Greco Roman and freestyle wrestling, sambo, boxing, kickboxing, Krav Maga, muay Thai, and Brazilian Jiu-Jitsu. Mark is a certified Arrest & Control Instructor with the Los Angeles Police Department and teaches at Jean Jacques Machado Brazilian Jiu-Jitsu Academy in Los Angeles. He also provides training though Mireles Combative Systems, a division of Mireles & Associates, a professional security consulting firm based in Burbank, CA.

Mark is a two-time recipient of the Medal of Valor, the highest award for bravery given by the LAPD and he was nominated for the Carnegie Medal, a prestigious award that honors extreme heroism to recipients in the United States and Canada. He has served in a variety of assignments including, patrol, narcotics, gangs, and career criminal apprehension. In addition to his field duties, Mark teaches police defensive tactics, officer safety, use-of-force policy, and investigative subject matters to police officers. Prior to his law enforcement career he served in the United States Marie Corps. Contact Mark at www.mirelespi.com.

Many thanks to Machado black belt Jamie Walsh for playing the attacker and to Sergeant Joe Klorman (LAPD) for his fine work behind the camera.

20 Ways to Hit and Grapple the Heavy Bags

By Loren W. Christensen

When you begin training in the martial arts and approach the heavy bag for the first time, you probably believe that punching the thing is simply a matter of slamming your fist into it. So, you hit it and that immediate shot of pain in your wrist and knuckles gives you pause, and the realization that there must be more to the bag than just whacking it. It's at this point that martial artists do one of two things: they don't hit it anymore or they buckle down and figure out how to master it.

Those who ignore it are taking a training path that is incomplete. Their power will never reach full potential and they will never understand the somewhat complex issues involved in hitting a solid mass that comes fairly close to duplicating a human. I'm not going to take the time to argue the merits of bag work because there is no argument. To repeat, training without bag work is incomplete training.

This chapter is for those fighters who believe in the merits of bag training, for those who followed up that first punching experience with lots of training. They have become quite skilled at punching and kicking it and have thus come full circle in their belief. They started out thinking that punching the thing is simply a matter of slamming your fist into it. Then they instantly discovered that there is more to it. They trained long and hard to master it and eventually returned to believing that punching the thing is simply a matter of slamming your fist into it.

This is similar to what Bruce Lee said about his training. "Before I studied the art, a punch to me was just like a punch, a kick just like a kick. After I learned the art, a punch was no longer a punch, a kick no longer a kick. Now that I've understood the art, a punch is just like a punch, a kick just like a kick."

Now let's take your bag training to a new place, to where punching and kicking it are no longer the same.

You're going to be fighting your heavy bag in ways that will look weird to the uninitiated peeping Tom peering through your window. You're going to punch the bag while lying on top of it, while lying underneath it, and while thrashing about with it. If you have ever seen those old Tarzan movies, the ones filmed back in the 1940s and 1950s on a backlot of a California movie studio, you saw the jungleman thrash about with a "lion" that was clearly a big stuffed doll. Then there was that crushing anaconda that was obviously a stuffed, uh, snakedoll. Remember how Tarzan flung it all about his body as he pretended to fight for his life? Well, that's what you're going to do, but with a heavy bag. You might feel strange at first (embarassed if the bag beats you) but keep at it to enjoy a whole new world of training possibilities.

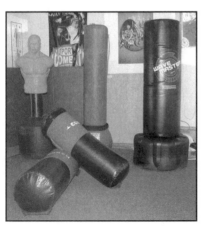

Stations

Let's begin by looking at a fun way to train using a variety of bags. In this case, I'm using the assorted bags that I have in my home training area, a two-car garage that I converted into a school several years ago. I've been able to aquire several kinds of bags over the years which allow me to practice different drills and exercises. This allows me to set up what I call "stations," where each bag is worked in a different manner for a given time limit. When I want to work aerobically, which is most of the time, I move through the stations nonstop, that is, I don't rest until the 20- or 30-minute session is over.

The good ol' 20- and 30-minute drills

If you have read my other books you know I favor 20- and 30-minute solo training workouts. While this is minimum for aerobic training, it nonetheless gives you a good training session that taxes your cardiovascular system and muscles. Do this two or three days on top of your regular training and you're on a quick path to fitness and fight preparedness.

If 20- and 30-minute sessions aren't enough for you, simply repeat as needed. Do the same drill again beginning at the same starting point as you just did, or start from the end and go through the drills ending at the first one. Or, design two or three 20- or 30-minute drills and flow from one to the other on those days you feel like a million bucks. But when you feel like a $1.42, just do one session.

How long at each station?

It's your workout so you decide. At first, I suiggest 5 minutes at each. If you have six stations, as I show here, 5 multiplied by six gives you a 30-minute workout. After three or four workouts, you might decide that you need more time at, say, one of the grappling stations. This is doable. Simply alter your session so that you grapple on the floor with the big bag for 10 minutes and then spend 4 minutes at each of the other five stations.

How intense?

Depends on how you feel. You feel like a million bucks? Go hard. You feel like $1.42? Go easy. You start out feeling one way and then it changes in the middle of the workout? Then change your intensity in the middle, too.

This happens a lot. You start out full of vim and vigor and 15 minutes into your session it's as if someone pulled the plug on your energy. If it's clearly physical – be careful because sometimes your mind can play games – then slow down. Continuing to go hard on just your nerve endings is not only unhealthy, it's dangerous and can lead to injury. Other times, working out is the last thing you want to do but you drag yourself to your training area - darn that discipline! – and voila! 15 minutes into your slow session you feel like a superhero. Take advantage of the moment and kick up your training a few nothches to enjoy a hard workout.

What should you do?

If this concept is new to you, follow the workout listed here. Follow it for a while until you get a feel for an area where you need more training or you find something that you really enjoy and want to do more of it. You only have so much energy so you will probably want to cut one station and double the time on another. Modify it however you want. What follows is the routine I've been doing for the past couple of weeks.

Okay, you've stalled enough. Let's get reeeeady to solo rumble!

Mannequin-style bag – neck attack

This session is to get you to think about the neck as a powerful target in your self-defense arsenal. So that is your only target as you hit and grapple it non-stop for 5 minutes. Do single hits and short and long combos. Flow from hitting to choking and from choking to hitting. Use the same concept to attack only the eyes or only the nose.

- Uppercut his throat

- Elbow to the side of the neck

- Chop the sides

- Forearm slam his Adam's apple

- Elbow the back of his neck

- Carotid constriction from the side

- Hammer the side of the neck

- Windpipe choke from the rear

- Forearm slam his brachial plexus

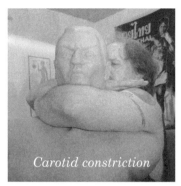

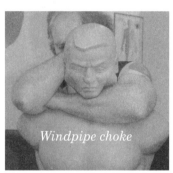

Carotid constriction

Windpipe choke

Heavy bag on the floor – hitting

I like to mix the intensity so that I hit 5-minutes on an "easy" station then move to 5 minutes on a harder one. For "easy," I started with the mannequin-style bag, which really isn't that easy when you push yourself to go hard and fast. But it's easier than this session where you're on the floor and hitting the bag, which represents a downed opponent. Anytime you're on the floor and thrashing around with a havy bag you're burning calories at an accelerated rate and huffing like a steam locomotive going up hill.

I have two portable heavy bags, a smaller one and a larger one. I use the smaller one for this drill since it's all about hitting as opposed to rolling around with it. I use the heavier one later in the rolling around session.

The bag is down and you're on it. You're going to throw straight punches, hook punches, claws, hammer strikes, elbows, head butts, knees, heel kicks, and run over it with a lawn mower. Just kidding about the last one, but the idea is to hit it with your arsenal to see what you can and can't do very well. An extreme example of the latter would be a spinning backfist. You can't do it while lying on the floor, at least not very well.

If you have experience hitting a downed bag, then simply go at whatever intensity you have used before. But if this is new to you, proceed cautiously until you get a feel for hitting downward as opposed to throwing blows at an upright target. For example, I get a major headache when elbowing the bag in the prone, but I don't when standing. I'm hoping it will pass but so far it hasn't. So I hit at about 75 percent for now. You would be wise to hit at 75 percent intensity, or less, until you get a sense for your techniques.

Do 1 set of 10 reps of all the following within 5 minutes.

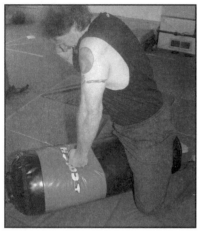

Straddle the bag and throw 20 alternating straight punches into it.

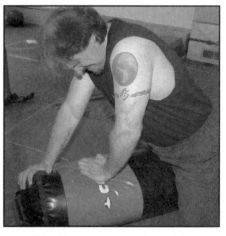

Straddle the bag and bend forward, leaning one hand on it. Throw 10 palm-heel punches with your other. Switch and do 10 reps on the other side.

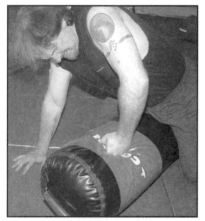

Straddle the bag. Bend forward with one hand on the floor and throw 10 straight punches. Switch and do 10 reps on the other side.

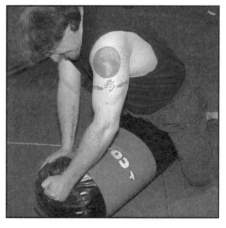

Straddle the bag and lean one hand on it. Slam it with hammerfist strikes. Switch and do 10 reps with your other arm.

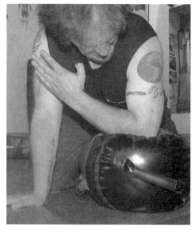

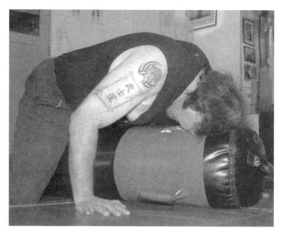

Straddle the bag. Bend forward and lean one hand on the floor, and throw elbow strikes into it. Switch and do 10 reps with your other arm.

Straddle the bag. Place both hands on the floor and headbutt the bag.

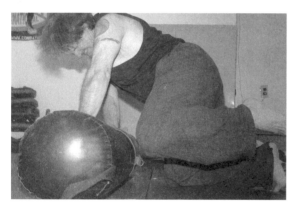

Face the bag from the side, place both hands on it and slam it with your knees.

Heavy bag - hit and grapple

In this station, you get to hit and grapple, that is, grapple within the limitations of the bag's design. It's a step above pantomining grappling techniques in the air and a step below grappling with a live person. But when you can't get a real partner or you just want to practice hitting harder and slamming a grappling technique on harder than what a live person would condone, the heavy bag is your ticket.

329

This station can be done on a hanging bag or a free standing one as I'm using in the pic. The primary difference is that when working on a hanging bag, you have to move from your hit to your grappling technique quickly before it swings too far away. As always, experiment to see what you can and cannot do. Here are a few ideas.

Clinch, palm-heel to the face, and shoot for the knees:

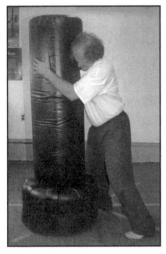

You're clinching the bag.

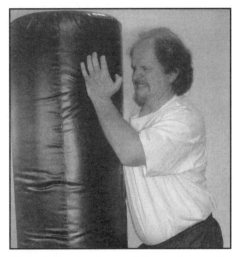

Slam it in the face with a palm strike.

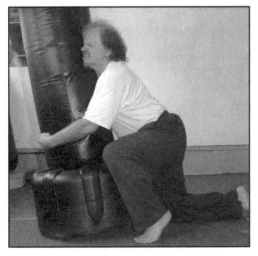

Shoot down to yank the knees and simultaneously slam your shoulder at groin level.

Block, elbow strike and bear hug:

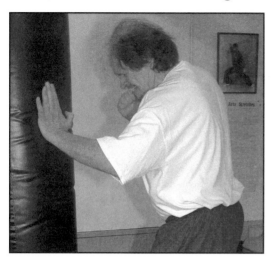

Imagine the threat launches a right punch at you. Slam your open hand against the side of the bag to simulate a sweep block.

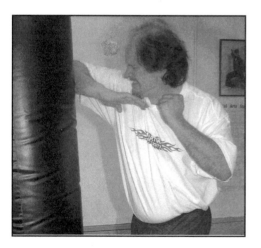

Follow with a right elbow smash at neck or face level.

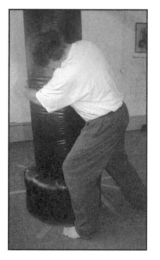

Step a little to the left to simulate moving to the threat's side and then wrap your arms around its ribs and crush. From here you would throw him onto his back or drive him into furniture.

Hit and clothesline:

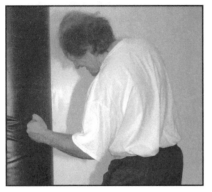 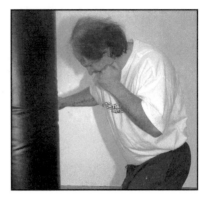

Slam in two hard hook punches, a lead arm...   .... and a rear arm.

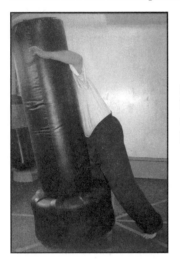

Slam the bag high with a stiff, but slightly bent left arm as if impacting the attacker's throat. Take a step past the bag to simulate knocking him to the ground.

Double-end bag – claws, rakes, pokes

Clearly this isn't a heavy bag but I insert it here to have 5 minutes in which I can get my breath back from the previous stations and let my heart rate return to where it's not trying to punch it's way out of my skin.

Clawing the double-end bag is about foot work, body and head evasion, and quick hands. You don't have to line up as precisley as is required when punching the bag because you're simply scraping and ripping it with your claws. It doesn't have to swing out and back on a straight track, which is often the case when punching. In fact, with this exercise, you want the bag to flip flop all over the place.

Think in terms of ripping the adversary's face and eyes as opposed to slamming his head with power. This gives you more freedom to impact the bag from any position. You can rake it as it comes directly at you, as it passes by your shoulder, and even after it has passed completely by. All that is required is quick footwork and body movement to keep the bag from slamming you.

Smack the bag so it begins to swing.

- Claw, rake or poke it with one hand as it swings back.

- Claw, rake, or poke it with two hands as it swings back.

- Sidestep and claw, rake, or poke it as it passes.

- Sidestep and claw, rake, or poke it as it returns.

- Lunge and claw, rake or poke.

- Chase and claw, rake or poke.

- Duck and claw, rake, or poke.

- Stop it with one hand and claw, rake or poke it with the other

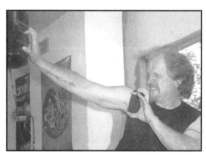

Claw, rake or poke the bag

Grappling and hitting the heavy bag on 4 sides

Don't practice this station after eating a chili burger because you're going to be panting and puffing hard as you thrash around with the heaviest bag you have. If you're already versed with training on a floor bag, insert your routine here for 5 minutes. If you aren't then use mine.

This session is especially beneficial if you're a karate, taekwondo or kung fu student because the close proximity of the bag – actually you're lying on top of it or it's lying on top of you, places you outside of your comfort zone. Sometimes you're in a position to hit and sometimes you're not. So when you aren't, what are you going to do?

You're going to start on top of the bag, then roll with it onto your left side, then roll with it onto your back with the bag on top of you, then roll with it onto your right side, and then roll once more until you're on top of it again. In each of these four positions you're going to fight the bag doing everything to it but pushing it away from you (if you push it away it makes for a short exercise). Hit it in whatever way you can and grapple using any technique that fits the moment. Clearly you can't do finger locks or toe twist, so you're going to have be creative, just as you would on the street should the assailant be wearing heavy winter gloves and boots.

Since the session is 5 minutes long and there are only four sides to the exercise, here are two options to burn up that extra minute.

Hit and grapple for 1 minute and 15 seconds on each side. That is the easy way or, rather, the easiest of the two options. Another 15 seconds in each position will seem like a half hour until you get into top shape.

The harder way is to repetitiously pick the bag up to shoulder height and then drop or slam it to the floor. Lifting the bulky, heavy and awkward weight will build your strength differently than an exercise machine where you must follow a given track. Lifting human weight isn't anything like working on an exercise machine. The bag comes pretty close to lifting the awkwardness that is a person, except it doesn't punch you in the face when you lift it off it's "feet." Lift it up and slam it down, then do it again.

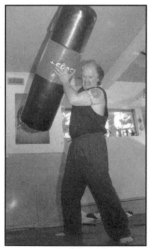

First minute: Bend down, pick up the bag and lift, using your knees to save your back to lift another day. Hoist it up onto your shoulder or, at arm's length overhead if you're feeling especially strong, and then drop it or slam it to the floor. Bend down and scoop it up again. Repeat for 1 minite. Shoot for 15 reps.

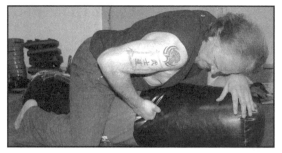

Second minute: After dropping the bag the last time, straddle it like a bronco rider in a rodeo. Without hesitation, pummel it with hooks, straight punches, elbows, forearms and head butts. Go for 1 minute.

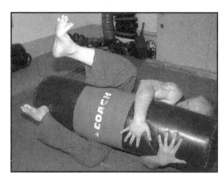 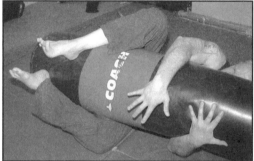

Third minute: Hold onto the bag with your arms and legs and roll over onto your left side. Heel kick the lower portion of the bag with your top leg. Scissor it with both and squeeze. You're hugging the bag now so your hitting options are reduced. Try elbows, headbutts, finger claws. What else can you do? Experiment and see.

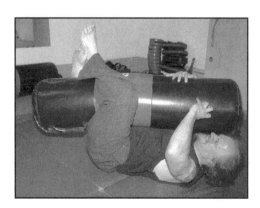

Fourth minute: At the end of the third minute, roll onto your back, hugging the bag. Claw the face, gouge the eyes. Wrap your arms into a fat-neck headlock and scissors the lower portion of the bag with your legs and squeeze at both ends. Headbutt. Bite (you might want to simulate). Hammer strike it. Slam it with your forearms. Experiment with what you can and can't do.

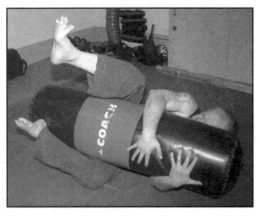

Fifth minute: At the end of the last minute, roll onto your right side. The situation here is basically the same as it was in the third minute. You're hugging the bag so your hitting options are reduced. Try elbows, headbutts, finger claws. Heel kick the lower portion of the bag with your top leg, scissor it with both, and squeeze. Experiment and then experiment some more

Heavy stationary bag – isometric push

The bag has to be stationary because you're pushing against it in an isometric exercise fashion, that is, pitting all your strength agaist it for a moment. If you only have a mannequin bag, position it at its lowest setting and lower your stance so you impact it close to the base. The closer you are to it's heavy foundation, the more stable it is. If you don't have a statioary bag, you will have to get help from a partner, which, of course, takes the solo aspect out of this exercise. Maybe the two of you can do stations together and help each other with this phase of it.

The idea is to punch the bag but not snap your hand back. Instead, press your fist into the bag as hard as you can at impact. I like pressing for 5 seconds, sometimes up to 10. If you do it that long, I suggest doing this phase of stations at the end of your workout as it's an energy and strength drainer. If you just press for one second, which is an option, you can do this station anywhere in your routine.

Your objective here is to strenghen your focus muscles, all those involved with tensing your strike at the moment of impact. I'm particularly fond of this exercise and find that I get a muscle pump from it, primarily in my shoulders, triceps and chest. Mostly, though, it has dramatically increased the power of my straight punches, hooks, and backfist.

Here is my current routine. All techniques are fired from a forward stance. All the pressing is done at maximum intensity.

- Straight punch and push for 5 seconds.10 reps both arms.

- Double punch and push for 5 seconds. 10 reps both arms.

- Hook punch and push for 5 seconds. 10 reps both arms.

- Double hook punch

  o Execute a rear-hand hook and press for 5 seconds

  o Execute a left hook punch as you retract the first one. Press for 5 seconds.

  o Do 10 reps then switch to your other leg forward. Do another 10 reps, pressing each one for 5 seconds.

- Backfist and press for 5 seconds. 10 reps both arms.

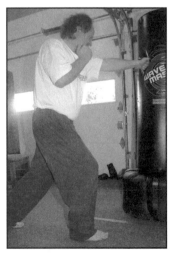
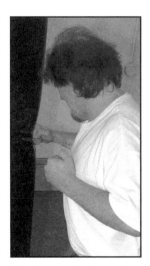
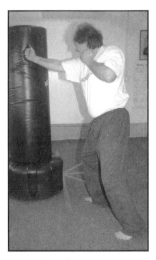

Straight punch & push   Hook punch & push   Backfist & press

Standing in place as you punch and kick the heavy bag is a viable, but basic concept within the box. You want to think outside the box. The more you play with the bags and unleash your imagination, the more ideas you will find that you can incorporate into your workouts

*L*oren W. Christensen's biography appears in the "About the Author" page at the back of the book.

Thanks to Lisa Christensen for her photography.

GRAPPLING

12 Ways to Attack the Hair

By Loren Christensen

Every cop has his bread-and-butter techniques, moves that he does fairly well and that work for him consistently. Some like armbars, others like foot sweeps, and some of them big ol' Texas boys like to simply overpower bad guys with their mass.

I liked to pull hair. I don't agree that it's girly fighting, as some people have argued. I use it to inflict excruciating pain, to apply leverage, and to give direction, usually onto the floor or into a wall. It works 95 percent of the time, a claim few techniques can make. If the awful pain doesn't stop an adversary from fighting you and force him to comply with your wishes, the leverage advantage you get when pulling from a high place makes it hard for him to physically continue. Mainly because he is too busy falling down.

War story

My partner and I got a radio call to assist another police car at a family fight, a type of call that is often quite dangerous to officers. Usually it's husband vs. wife, mother vs. daughter, or father vs. son. The battle reaches such intensity that someone calls 9-1-1 and, into that inferno, the cops must go, sometimes to get whacked by a frying pan or stabbed with garden shears. This time though the situation was different: the danger wasn't to the cops.

We could hear the woman's screams from within the house as we sprinted up the stairs toward the open front door. They weren't screams of rage, so typical at a family fight. These were screams of panic.

"Pull him off! Pull him off!" the hysterical woman screamed as the four of us burst through the door. She stood bent over a sofa yanking on the arm of a man who lay face down on the cushions. "My baby!" she screeched.

It took a couple of seconds for the scene to make sense, for the horror of it to sink in. The man was lying on a baby attempting to suffocate it with his chest. Judging by the tiny purple foot and leg that extended oddly out from under the man's armpit, he was succeeding.

The closest officer struck the man in the head with his fist, as did his partner. But the man only squeezed tighter. Again they struck him, and my partner tried to pull his arms out from under him. All to no avail.

I plunged my right hand into the man's bushy hair all the way to his scalp, and twisted it as far as I could, about 180 degrees. Still he wouldn't let go. So with my left hand I grabbed the same hair from where I had twisted it with my right, and rotated it another 180, ripping it from his scalp by the dozens, probably by the hundreds. The assailant screamed, and with one arm pushed himself up from the cushions and off the baby, as his other arm reached desperately toward the agony at the top of his head.

The baby lay silently, motionless. Then it screamed bloody murder. He was alive and pretty darn mad. One of the officers grabbed him before he rolled off the sofa's edge.

I yanked the man's hair forward so that he fell back onto the sofa and then jerked it hard to side to fling him to the floor. I admit I twisted his hair with every ounce of strength I had and I further admit that for a moment there my professional neutrality waned. Two of the other officers wrenched his arms behind his back and secured his wrists with handcuffs.

In the end, the man was able to tolerate the officers' desperate head punches but not the pin-point agony of his hair twisted so hard it ripped from his scalp in bunches.

Acute pain and direction

Pain

The beauty of hair pulling, that is, the beauty from the standpoint of the one executing the move, is that while the techniques are acutely painful, they hurt only during their application. Release the hold and the pain stops. It doesn't leave a mark on the recipient's body, no evidence for him to later photograph and then hire an attorney to sue because you hurt him. The pain stops when you release the hold. If you're left holding a few hairs, simply dust your hands off into the wind.

To say that the pain is acute is an understatement. When you do the technique correctly, it feels to your recipient as if his scalp were being ripped from his skull. The pain is sharp and deep and even the heavily intoxicated feel it.

Direction

I prefer grappling techniques that give direction, meaning that the pain or leverage directs the recipient into a wall, over a coffee table, or down to the floor. In my experience, techniques that hurt but don't direct, have a greater potential to prolong the fight, antagonize the assailant, and cause him greater injury. Hair techniques give clear direction, specifically, away from the pain. Should the confrontation end up in court, you can tell the jury that though there were other techniques you could have applied, you chose hair techniques because they give clear direction and are likely to end the confrontation quickly without causing injury.

Now, the jury probably won't hoist you onto their shoulders and carry you out of the courtroom chanting your name in adoration, but they will understand that you didn't want to prolong or seriously hurt the person who attacked you. That is a good thing in the eyes of the law.

Bald guys

I have yet to teach a hair technique class without someone raising their hand and asking, "What if the guy is bald? Can you still do hair techniques on him?"

Amazingly, there are always a couple of other people nodding to show that they were wondering the same thing.

Now, there is an axiom in teaching that says: "There is no such thing as a stupid question."

I disagree.

Tolerance

Sometimes intoxicated, high, and mentally deranged people are tolerant to the pain of hair techniques. I've also noticed that some women react differently than most men. I found this to be true even in class where the adrenaline level is lower than in a street fight.

I know of no studies as to why some women don't feel hair techniques as intensely as men. It could be because they have a higher tolerance to pain or perhaps it's because some women brush their hair every night for the mandatory 200 strokes to bring on that desired luster. Over time, this makes the nerves around their hair follicles less vulnerable to pain. Okay, that theory might not be the best, but until someone gets a million dollar government grant and conducts a study, I'm running with it.

There are two ways to fix this problem. First, be sure to reach into a woman's hair far enough for your fingers to scrape the scalp as you gather hair. Then ball your hand into a tight fist. This ensures that you're pulling and twisting at the scalp level as opposed to out toward the ends of her hair. Second, if you grab correctly and the woman isn't reacting to the pain, immediately change the technique to a leverage move. More on this in a moment.

Female fights on video Have you ever watched any of the many Hollywood "news" television programs where they show footage of celebrities acting badly? The shows frequently show video taken by the paparazzi of a couple of young female stars fighting in a parking lot. Quite often, the two are yanking each other's hair as they scream and thrash about. However, rarely is the hair pulling causing the women pain. This is because the pullers are always gripping the ends of the hair rather than reaching deeply to the scalp. On the positive side for the puller, the receiver usually goes in the direction in which the hair is pulled. It's the old adage: *Where the head goes the body follows.*

Elements that make hair techniques work

Here are a few elements that dramatically increase your success rate when using hair techniques.

Where to grab:

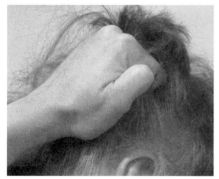

You must clench your fist deeply into the hair to grasp at the roots.

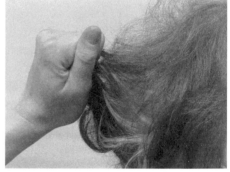

Grabbing at the ends makes for an insecure hold and delivers little pain.

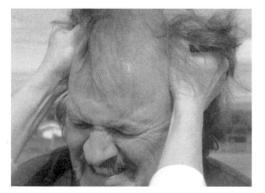

Grabbing the hair on the sides of the head is more painful than on top of the head.

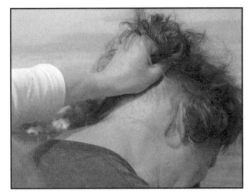

Grabbing at the back of the head, close to the neck where the hairs are shorter and more sensitive, gives you great control of the adversary. Rotate your hand left, he goes left. Rotate it right, he goes right. Sort of like piloting an airplane but with screams and curses.

To apply pain:

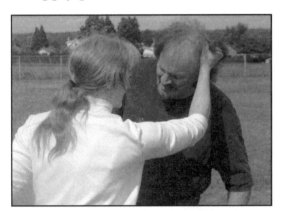

Bad pain: Jerk your hand in whatever direction you choose. Remember that he will follow his hair, so if you jerk your hand toward your chest he will slam into you.

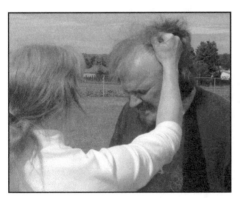
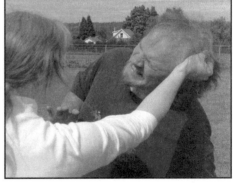

Super pain: Twist your hand with a snapping motion (as if turning a doorknob quickly) clockwise or counterclockwise.

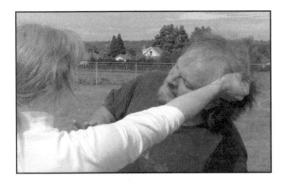

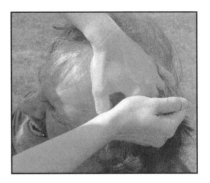

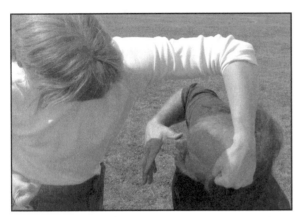

Nasty pain: Twist with a snapping motion as far as you can with one hand. Then insert your other hand where your first hand ended its rotation and continue to twist the hair even farther.

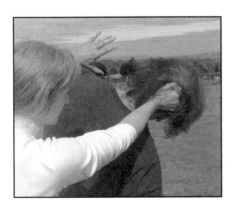

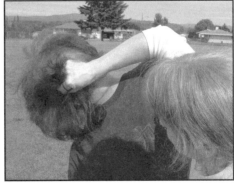

Excruciating pain: Jerk and twist your hand in one direction and then without hesitation jerk and twist your hand in another direction.

To upset his balance:

Grab a wad of hair.

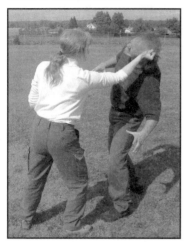 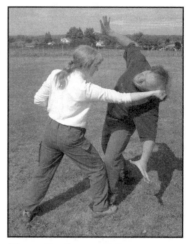

Pull or twist it so the adversary
leans heavily on one leg.

Trap the leg and dump
him on the ground.

Grab the sides of his head from the front with both hands.

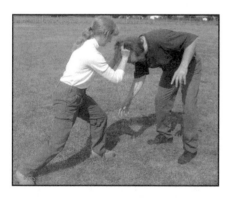 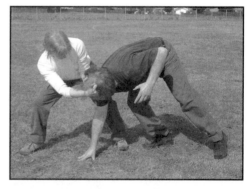

Tuck your elbows hard toward the
ground.

Step back to give him room to fall.

Grab his hair at the back of his head.

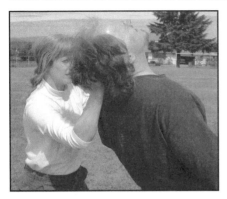

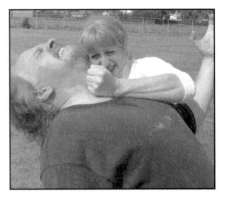

Pull him backwards by tucking your elbow toward the ground.

Hammerfist his face or neck as you pull him to the ground.

To finish him off:

You have secured the hair on the sides of his head.

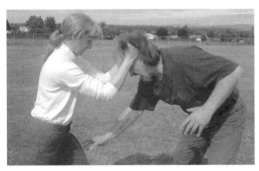

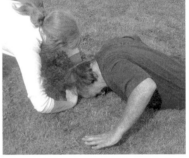

Twist your hands forward and tuck your elbows to pull him down.

Keep hold of his hair as he sprawls on his chest

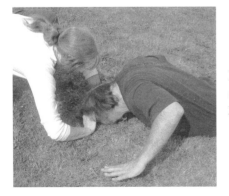

If he begins to push himself up, sharply rotate your hands toward you and slam his face into the ground.

Two painful takedowns:

From behind the adversary, grab the hair on both sides of his head.

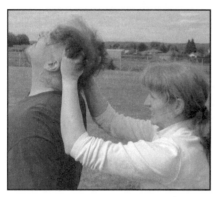

Rotate your hands toward you and tuck your elbows.

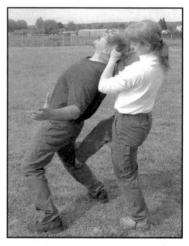

Should you have problems, kick behind his knee to buckle his legs.

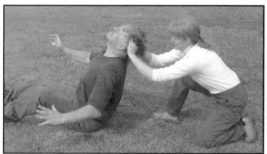

He will land on his rear or back.

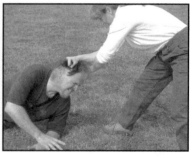

Push one hand up and over and push the other down and under...

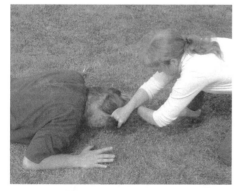

...to force him painfully over onto his belly. This crossed arm position is a tad awkward so when the moment is right either switch hand positions and continue to restrain using his hair, or stand up and run.

Grab the sides of the adversary's head from the front.

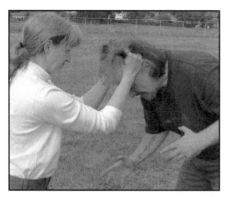

Rotate your hands toward you and tuck your elbows.

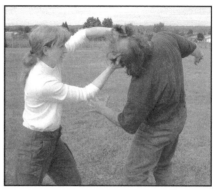

When he is half way down, abruptly swoop your arms (and his head) to the right or left...

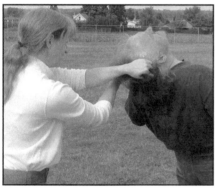

...until your arms are crossed and the adversary is bent over backwards.

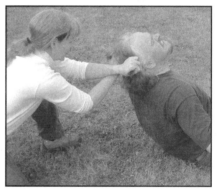

Pull his hair downward so he falls onto his back.

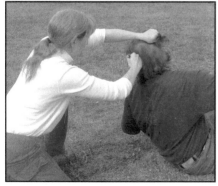

Immediately, forcefully uncross yours arms...

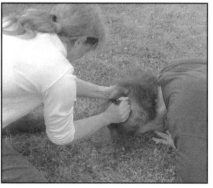

...so that he flips over onto his back. Twist downward to restrain him.

Potential problems

Here are a few problems I've had when doing hair techniques or that have been reported back to me.

- It's hard to grip greasy hair.

- Some people, because of poor diet, alcoholism, or illness lose their hair in chunks when pulled.

- Some wigs look realistic, so much so that you will be left standing holding one as the balding assailant runs off or attacks you even angrier than before.

- It is potentially injurious to your fingers. I have sprained mine trying to control especially violent people and I know of one police officer who broke his, leaving it permanently deformed.

- Some people hide weapons in their hair, such as razorblades.

- Pulling someone's hair is likely to enrage that person's friends and even uninvolved people. For reasons that aren't always clear, hair pulling can evoke anger in third party observers.

- There is a potential that you could injure an adversary's neck by jerking him about by his hair. So use caution and be justified.

Hair techniques hurt. They aren't even fun to practice because they hurt so much. (Nor was it fun doing this photo shoot. I was hurting for several hours after.) They hurt when you first grab a handful next to the scalp and the pain increases when you pull, twist, yank, and rotate it.

I highly recommend them.

Loren **W. Christensen**'s biography appears in the "About the Author" page at the back of the book.

Thanks to Lisa Christensen (sort of) for her (over) exuberant work pulling my hair, and to Amy Widmer for her work behind the camera.

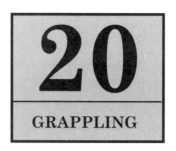

5 Ways to Apply Carotid Constriction
The Street Fighter's Magic Punch

by Mark Mireles

The mystical aspects of the martial arts are appealing to many Western students, such as the power of chi, supernatural strength, lightning-fast reactions, and blue lightNing bolts coming from a master's eyes. Often when I teach classes and give seminars, a student will ask me what is the one unstoppable technique that never fails. I tell him that there is no such thing and what he is really looking for is a shortcut. But there are none. It's not his fault; after all he is at the beginning of a very long journey.

The term "magic punch" refers to that so-called mystical technique. Yes, it's meant pejoratively, but I use it here to make the point that there is no magic punch. But boy, do we all wish there were. It would be the fast food of the martial arts, and whether that's good or bad we will never know for there is only hard work and relentless training on the path to learning.

But wait. One technique comes close to fitting the magic punch definition because when used properly by a skilled person the technique indeed does appear to be magical. I'm referring to the art and science of mastering carotid constriction.

Versatile problem solver

Pick a martial arts magazine off the newsstand or browse the latest martial arts selection at the bookstore and you will see something about carotid constriction, sometimes known as sleeper holds. Martial artists agree that it's a powerful method of attack and defense.

The unique benefits of carotid constriction include:

- The technical aspects of carotid constriction don't rely on great physical strength.

- It doesn't matter if your attacker is high on drugs or alcohol.

- It doesn't matter if your attacker is displaying superhuman strength.

There are many methods of applying carotid constriction, but there are only two schools: constriction using clothing and constriction without it. There is debate between some martial artists as to which method is better. I have trained in both methods and, in my humble opinion, I have found that both are of value on the street, especially since you never know what your attacker will be wearing or in what environment or weather condition you will be doing battle.

The art and science of carotid constriction

Applying a constriction technique is both art and science. The systematic application of a technique is the science portion of correct carotid constriction, what I call the easy part since a monkey could learn the strictly physical aspects. What makes the technique truly effective in hand-to-hand combat is the art aspect.

The art of the technique occurs when after learning the move you then apply your personal signature. It begins with an understanding of your own physical make-up, your level of ability, and then returns full circle to that of applying your intellect. The art of fighting is the "you" behind the scientific principles. Your trained ability is what moves a technique from a strict science to an art

Carotid constriction defined

The definition of carotid constriction for our purposes is:

- a control hold that uses your arms to apply a lock around the neck of an attacker. When you apply sufficient pressure to the carotid arteries on one or both sides of the neck, it renders the person unconscious.

- a control hold in which you manipulate the attacker's clothing, usually the collar, to apply pressure against the carotid arteries, thus rendering him unconscious.

These two methods constrict the blood flow to the brain. Without a sufficient blood supply, the brain goes to sleep. When the technique is correctly applied, the attacker loses consciousnes in 8 to 15 seconds.

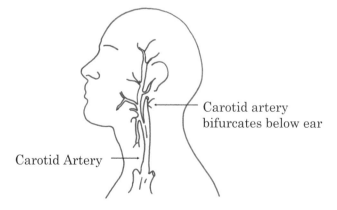

Carotid artery
bifurcates below ear

Carotid Artery

The two carotid arteries —one on each side of the neck - carry oxygen-rich blood away from the heart to the brain. Pressure applied to one or both arteries will render the person unconsciousness. *(Illustration by Kris Wilder)*

form. That is what separates you from the monkeys.

Fighting is similar to a game of chess. The successful martial artist stays two or three steps ahead of his opponent so that he can checkmate. As a martial artist, you need to be able to impose your mental strengths, a process that takes time to develop. It's a place where the body and mind become connected and a place where you feel the situation unfolding like a chess master sees an opening on the board. Dedicated practice eventually makes this thought process very short.

Concepts based training

Here is a phenomenon that often occurs in martial arts training. A new student in a sterile environment learns a technique that is broken down for him into steps 1, 2 and 3, which eventually he can do flawlessly with a partner. Later, however, when the moment of truth arrives in the form of a street fight, the technique doesn't work. He does step 1, step 2, and *Bang!,* the student gets counter pummeled. The magic punch failed! Once he stops seeing stars, he is shocked that his training didn't work. This leads to self-doubt and the self-doubt expands to doubting the fighting system. Either the student quits training or he goes in search of the Holy Grail of a fighting art elsewhere. In reality, the problem isn't the technique at all. The problem is that it wasn't trained realistically.

When it comes to any martial arts training there has to be adequate explanation of how and when to apply techniques. The problem with the above training scenario is that it only covered the mechanics of the technique, the how. This is important in the initial phase of instruction but then the student must learn the practical application/reality phase, too.

Concepts should be the foundation of a fighting system that form a cycle that your training must ingrain in you. There are three concepts related to carotid constriction:

- Control
- Positioning
- Entry

Control and positioning

To apply a constriction technique, you first have to control your opponent and then establish a dominant position. Control and position are closely related but they are not the same thing. In the example of our frustrated student, he lacked the control and positioning segments of the concepts. He had learned the mechanics, but he didn't learn how to apply the technique against someone fighting back.

Look at the photos in any old judo text to see an example of what I'm talking about. The attacker appears in an almost formal position applying the constriction technique on the defender who is in an equally formal but cooperative position. The author explains the techniques fully in the text but the antecedents - position and control - are missing. Real fighting is explosive and your training needs to reflect this dynamic to be effective on the street.

You can't learn to swim on dry land

The ability to control your opponent is a matter of hard physical training on your feet and on the ground. To learn the physics that control grappling, you need to be familiar with such fighting arts as judo, wrestling, sambo, and Brazilian jiu-jitsu. There is no substitute for actually getting out there and grappling all-out. Sign up for three months of grappling, get into a workshop, or participate in a few seminars. You're not looking to become an expert; you just want to be exposed to grappling systems to obtain a good base of knowledge.

I recommend exploring all the above systems to get as much information as you can from different instructors. Though the systems are all different, I like to think of them as cousin arts, as they all have good points. In particular, their live sparring sessions will give you the feel of a resisting opponent as you learn to control him.

Entry   Once you learn to control an opponent you will be able to get into dominant positions that allow you to execute constriction techniques. From the dominant position, the execution of the technique is called the "entry," the mechanics of the technique you're using to strangle.

Reality: sports vs. street fighting

I began martial arts training in 1977 at the age of 10 in a small dojo in the San Francisco Bay Area. Over the years, I have studied all forms of combative sports, and because of my profession, I have studied police defensive tactics and armed forces hand-to-hand combat. Allow me to draw on my background to make one point crystal clear: There is a galactic difference between street fighting and combative sports. Failure to recognize that fact could result in you sustaining serious injury, or worse. I know because I've been there.

I competed for many years in both judo and wrestling, but when I became a police officer, I found myself suddenly thrust into a world of extreme violence, *real* violence. In those early incidents, I came to a realization that the techniques I had learned in combative sports needed modification if I were to use them in real fighting. And that's exactly what I did.

For several years, the streets of Los Angeles became my laboratory. I modified what I learned in combative sports, incorporated new methods of street fighting, and evaluated the effectiveness of it all. I still enjoy wrestling gym wars and judo sparring in the dojo, but through experience, I understand that street fighting is an entirely different animal.

Positive crossovers

Combative sports are fine as long as you realize and remember that real fighting isn't a sport. Sports have rules while real fighting does not. There are no time limits on the street or a referee to stop the action. That said, combat sports do have several positive crossovers to real fighting.

- The mental toughness ingrained by physically demanding combative sports is invaluable.

- Many of the techniques are already street effective or need only slight modification to make them so.

- All-out sparring gives you a feel for how opponents move.

Evaluate your practice

Practitioners who come from a background of less demanding combat sports (i.e. less physical contact) need to evaluate honestly the readiness of their system's street effectiveness. In real fighting, punches and kicks are free to land with maximum force to any target on the body. Sometimes the fights are at close quarters and other times they go to the ground. There are many scenarios in street fighting, and to make your martial arts training street effective, you have to take what you already know and expand it. That goes for using carotid constriction techniques in your street fighting arsenal.

Two considerations often ignored when training for the street

As a practitioner of both judo and Brazil jiu-jitsu, there are methods of carotid

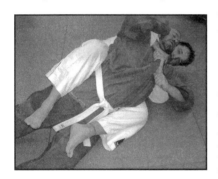

constriction and positions I use in class that I would never attempt on the street. For example, one chief difference between sports grappling and real fighting is the use of your legs to assist you in the application of carotid constriction. In sport grappling, you can use your legs to secure your opponent's legs while your arms apply the constriction technique.

But in a real fight you want to be mobile and use your feet to evade, kick, and run. Should you be fighting more than one person, you don't want to trade mobility for using your legs to tightly secure a carotid constriction technique. Multiple attackers are not a factor in the gym.

There is one other monumental factor. When applying a constriction technique on the street you have to consider that the opponent could have a weapon, even when he didn't present one in the initial stages of the fight. Weapons are a reality that you must always consider, especially since people can easily conceal handguns and knives, and then easily present them in close fighting.

That factor doesn't exist in the training hall; however, it isn't to be ignored in preparation for street combat.

The two-part mental game

First, is your ability to keep an open mind to facilitate learning and to quickly bridge the gap from training in combative sports to training for a real fight. It's a process of adjustment that is as much mental as it is physical. Fighting for sport is about winning trophies or money, while fighting on the street is about your personal protection and survival. If you're coming from a combat sports background or from an esoteric system that hasn't focused on the realities of street violence, you need to focus your mental processes on making the adjustment. You will make significant gains in your martial arts journey by keeping an open and positive mental state.

Second, you have to make up your mind that no matter how grave the conditions, you *will* survive. Every street fight is a life and death battle. While paranoia isn't part of a positive mental game plan, you don't have a crystal ball so your training must take into consideration the worst case scenarios. Start with making your training sessions tough. There are no short cuts so the effort you make in training relates directly to your martial arts effectiveness. Along with the tough training, you must develop a state of mind that *you will survive.*

Three methods of carotid constriction

Execute the following carotid constriction methods behind your opponent, meaning that your chest is against your attacker's back. This is a highly desirable position in real fighting because it reduces greatly your chance of getting stabbed or shot by an armed attacker.

Although the subject of police tactics and policy is beyond the scope of this writing, the methods cops learn are also relevant to your needs for street survival. As I tell my police students in defensive tactics classes, drugs and alcohol often numb the suspect's pain sensors but it doesn't improve the suspect's balance or protect the flow of blood to his brain. This makes constriction techniques the perfect option, simple moves predicated on surprise and quick application.

Most police officers in the United States learn the three carotid constraint techniques shown here, maneuvers based on the Japanese marital arts:

- Modified carotid control hold
- Full carotid control hold
- Lock carotid control hold

Field tested and humane

The law enforcement community is rich with master level martial artists who have been down dark alleys. These street veterans have taken what they have learned and applied it to what they encounter on the streets. Experience is worth its weight in gold. However, what really convinced me as to the effectiveness of law enforcement's techniques is that officers with no prior martial arts training are able to apply them successfully in field situations.

Police administrators have been supportive of carotid constriction holds because it's a humane defensive tactic. When a constriction hold is applied correctly, it renders an adversary unconscious, but it's not likely to injure him. That is important to you should you have to defend yourself for using it in criminal and civil court.

First, let's look at a simple way to get behind your opponent.

Shoulder smash

To apply the three variations, you must first establish control and position prior to entry. By using a technique called the shoulder smash, you employ the element of surprise to move from facing your opponent to taking control of his back. Practice the shoulder smash from both your right and left sides forward.

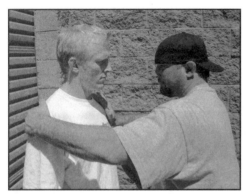

Palm strike his shoulder with one hand and pull his opposite shoulder with your other.

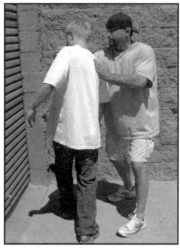

This forces your opponent to turn 180 degrees.

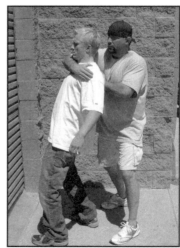

Once you have access to his back you can apply one of the following three upper body control holds.

Modified carotid control hold

Of the three upper body control holds, the modified carotid is the least effective. Consider this a transition position you apply after attacking with the shoulder smash. Generally, the modified carotid control hold doesn't put them to sleep as consistently as the other two methods, but it's still a valuable technique.

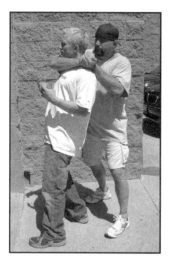

From behind your opponent, place your right arm around his neck. Center the inside of your elbow on the opponent's neck. Place your fisted hand into your cupped hand to form a lock around your opponent's neck.

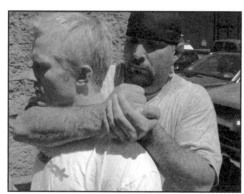

The crook of your right arm is under your opponent's chin.

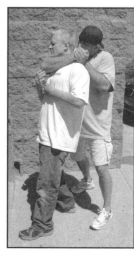

Apply pressure by pulling your fisted hand with your other hand. Apply additional pressure by attempting to press your elbows together.

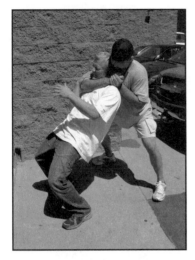

To take your opponent to the ground, simply take a small step backwards and, with maximum force, drive the elbow of your strangling arm toward the ground.

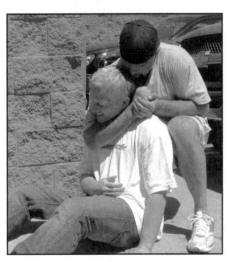

As your opponent sits, quickly evaluate the strength of your hold. Should he lose consciousness, you will feel him go limp, at which time you should immediately relax the hold but keep it in position. Should your opponent awaken and begin fighting again, quickly apply pressure again to send him to dream land.

Important point: When you feel your opponent's body go limp, relax the tension in your arms but don't give up the hold. He might be out for five seconds or 30; he might even be faking. Some awaken passive while others are even more combative. Should you disengage from the hold, you might have to apply the three-step control, positioning and entry all over again. Relax the pressure but keep your arms in place in case you have to apply the hold again or wait until help arrives.

The full carotid control hold

Once you have taken your opponent down with the modified carotid control hold, you can then flow into the full carotid control hold.

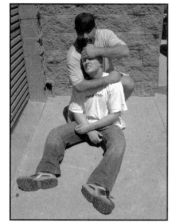

From the seated position, use the hand that was pulling the constricting hand to slap your opponent's forehead hard enough to knock his head back. This action opens his neckline and exposes both carotid arteries to allow you to transition into a very tight and full carotid control hold.

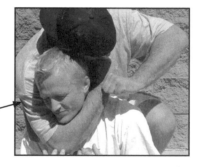

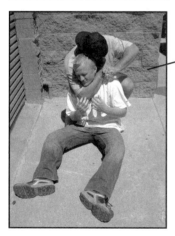

Your right bicep presses against the artery on the right side of his neck and your forearm presses against the left side. To make the hold even tighter, place the web of your left hand outside the wrist of your right hand. Then press your web against your wrist to create an ultra tight constriction.

Maintain a tight seal between the crook of the elbow and the neck to prevent him from tucking his chin to his chest to defeat your hold. Keep squeezing until you feel him go limp

Important point: Although you don't give up the hold once your opponent goes limp, it's critical to release the pressure immediately. **Should you continue to constrict his blood flow after he loses consciousness, you might cause brain damage or even death.** Release the pressure, but maintain a loose, no pressure hold.

The locked carotid control hold

This hold is an alternative to the full carotid control hold and is the most effective of all three. If the situation allows, this is the most desirable position of constriction because it's such an extreme hold.

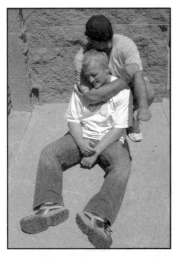

Place your right arm around your opponent's neck. Again, center the crook of your elbow in the middle of your opponent's chest. Place your right hand around your left biceps.

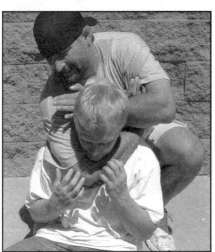

As you place your left arm behind your opponent's neck, your right thumb inserts tightly into your left armpit. The thumb position is hard to see in this photo but it's critical to the formation of a constricting neck hold. When your right thumb is in as deeply as possible, grip the biceps of your left arm tightly with your four remaining fingers.

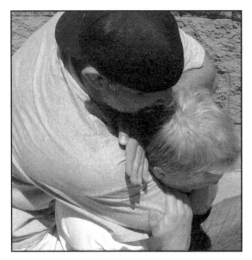

Your palm should face downward with your four fingers and thumb tight together. Your left hand resembles a karate chop.

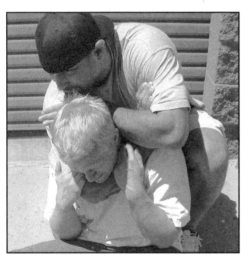

Compress the biceps of your right arm while driving your open left hand across your opponent's neck. The action of your arms resembles a scissors motion, one that constricts the blood supply to the brain. When you feel your opponent go limp, release the tension but keep the hold until you see what he is going to do.

Alternative to the locked carotid control hold   Instead of holding your left hand open hand behind your opponent's neck, grip your right shoulder to create a pressure hold.

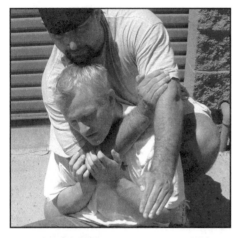

Grip your left biceps consistent with the above instructions.

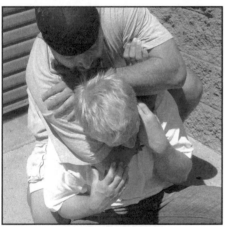

Again, insert your right thumb into your armpit and place your left arm behind your opponent's neck over the right arm. The difference in this version is that you cup your left hand over your right shoulder.

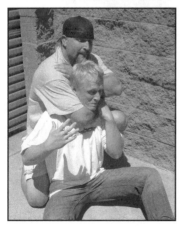

The hold becomes effective when you compress both biceps and forearms. This action creates a tight pressure lock constricting the blood supply to the carotid arteries. Relax the hold when you feel your opponent go limp and evaluate the situation. He may be playing possum.

Using the collar for constriction

During the dynamics of a street fight there are many opportunities to use the attacker's clothing as a weapon against him. A thick coat collar or sturdy shirt collar provides you two great handles for carotid constriction. Should your opponent be wearing a t-shirt, it's generally easier to just strangle the exposed neck as described in the last section. In addition, t-shirt material is generally unreliable and tears easily.

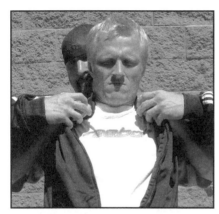

Secure both lapels under your opponent's arms and pull your elbows backward taking up the slack in his clothing.

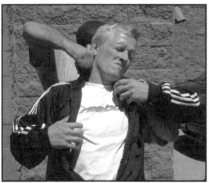

Place the knuckle of your right hand behind your attacker's ear.

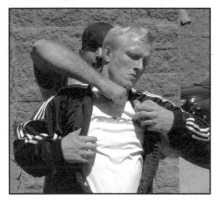

Slide your thumb knuckle along your attacker's jaw line.

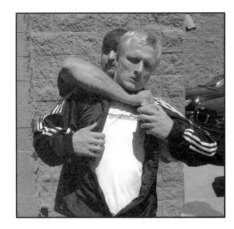

Then secure the opposite collar. Your left hand maintains a secure hold under the attacker's arm.

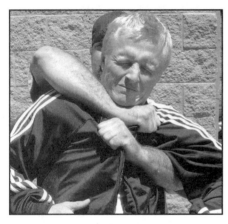

Then transition your left hand to secure the opposite collar to create a cross grip. Your left hand pulls downward on the opposite collar while your right hand pulls laterally across the shoulder line. This action constricts the brain's blood supply.

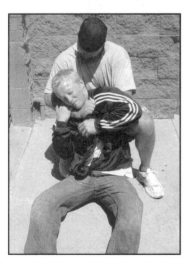

Step back to take him down as you did earlier. Unlike in sport grappling, only use your legs to secure your attacker's lower extremities as a last resort.

Carotid constriction counter measures

These three rules relate to you being on the receiving end of a carotid hold. Never break them.

Rule 1: Never give up your back   Never let your opponent get in back of you. This is an absolute whether you're fighting on your feet or on the ground. When your opponent gets behind you, applying a carotid constriction technique becomes an option for him.

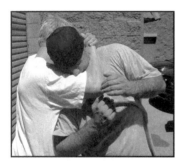

Rule 2: Protect your neckline   When your opponent attempts to strangle you, immediately protect your carotid arteries (also called the neckline). Do this by driving your chin into your chest.

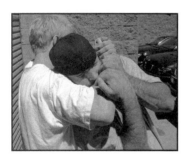

Rule 3: Never trust your neck   This means that you need to use your hands to block and break your opponent's lock on your neck. Though you have initially stymied the neck attack by driving your chin into your chest, he can still strangle you. You also need to get both your hands between your opponent's radius (wrist area) and your neck, and then pull his wrist downward.

Or, pull it downward and then push it upward over your face. It's hard to see in this position, so you need to feel your way to breaking the hold around your neck.

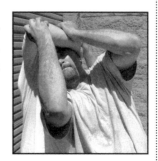

With good training, the above methods of constriction are effective and easy to do. Start slowly with your training partners with the goal to eventually applying the holds as they resist you. Practice with partners of various statures. A big person reacts different than does a wiry small person.

One final consideration is that of the legality of carotid constriction where you live. Self-defense and constriction techniques can be a tricky area in the law. This means that using these moves in self-defense could have a negative impact on you depending on how and where you use it. Know the laws where you live and understand the type of attack you're under. Using carotid constriction in a life-and-death situation is a different dynamic than using it against a drunk who pushes you in a bar.

In the end, you're going to do what you need to do to stay safe. Just remember that you will have to explain what happened, what prompted your actions, and why you chose to use a constriction. If you understand the laws and can speak intelligently about why you chose the self-defense option of carotid constriction, you will be in a better position. This is a critical factor often overlooked in martial arts training; it's unfortunate since we operate in a society of laws and sue-happy people.

Caution: Although carotid constriction holds are executed regularly in training and in competition with few injuries, several police agencies around the country have banned its use because people have died from it. Applying the constriction to a conditioned athlete who slaps out is one thing, but applying it to a drugged, intoxicated, or enraged person who continues to fight until he is unconscious is a different matter. Along with your knowledge of potentially lethal techniques, it's your responsibility to be certified in CPR, know the laws in your state as to using such lethal force, and know that you are legally obligated to call 911 should you seriously hurt someone.

Mark **Mireles**'s biography appears in Chapter 16, "The clinch for street fighting."

Many thanks to Machado black belt Jamie Walsh for playing the attacker and to Sergeant Joe Klorman (LAPD) for his fine work behind the camera.

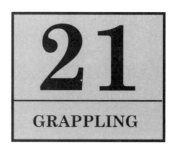

6 Ways to Use the Environment

Interview with Soke Tim Delgman, 9th dan
by Loren W. Christensen

Tim Delgman has been my friend and jujitsu teacher for many years. Besides his extraordinary knowledge of martial arts technique, history, and traditions, he is a gracious host and always willing to help and advise in my writing projects. Tim appears in several of my DVDs and never complains about the hard falls that he takes to make me look better than I am.

I sat with Soke Delgman and talked with him about aiki jujitsu and a few other things.

Loren W. Christensen (LWC): What is aiki jujitsu?

Tim Delgman (TD): Looking at the Japanese derivative, the letters "ai" means to coordinate, "ki" means breath or spirit, "ju" means gentle, and "jitsu" means art. Putting it all into context, aiki jujitsu is the "art of coordinating the spirit." However, we look at aiki as harmonizing. Thus, we harmonize in a gentle way.

Our founder, Professor Duke Moore, was a multi-talented person who knew multiple martial arts. The system incorporates elements of the grappling arts, boxing, and karate. I hesitate to say aikido and judo since those two martial arts are derivatives of jujitsu. Because of the incorporation of various martial arts within one system, we say that we coordinate various martial arts into a harmonious gentle art.

LWC: What is Zen Budo Kai Aiki jujitsu?

TD: Zen has a religious connotation that states that one can attain enlightenment through meditation, self-contemplation, and intuition, and a non-religious connotation meaning "all encompassing." "Budo" means martial way, "kai" means society, "aiki" means encompassing, "ju" means gentle, and "jitsu" means art. Thus loosely translated, Zen Budo Kai Aiki Jujitsu is the "all contemplating warrior society encompassing a gentle art." Professor Moore, however, translated it as "moving meditation." We like to think of ourselves as a society or club that learns and teaches a variety of martial arts for self-defense.

LWC: How is it different from Brazilian jujitsu? Is Brazilian jujitsu better than Japanese jujitsu? If not, why does the Brazilian system get so much attention?

TD: Brazilian jujitsu gained its notoriety from the Ultimate Fighting Championships (UFC), the sport made popular by the Gracies because they won so many tournaments. The basic idea in the UFC was to get the opponent to the ground and strangle him. Brazilian jujitsu is effective in the ring, but on the streets where you are likely to have more than one opponent, some consider it not as practical. My understanding is while Brazilian jujitsu came from Japan, the Brazilians put more emphasis on mat techniques.

Zen Budo Kai Aiki Jujitsu incorporates various martial arts. Although we do mat techniques, the emphasis in Zen Budo Kai Aiki Jujitsu is the blending of joint locking techniques and throws. Some of my students who have studied both systems feel that ours is more street oriented.

LWC: We have always heard that you don't have to be large and muscular to do jujitsu, but most of the grappling fighters on the circuit are obviously weight trained. Why is that?

TD: Judo, which means "the gentle way," is a sport designed for competition. The first thing these gentle people do is strengthen themselves with weights and aerobic exercise. They toughen themselves. If you are competing in any sport you should be in your best physical shape for that sport, whether it is wrestling, running, boxing or whatever. The grappling arts are no different, especially when you know you're competing with top individuals.

It's unlikely that tournament grapplers will attack you in the street. In the street, the average person who knows jujitsu will face the average person who knows street techniques. The goal in learning jujitsu is to take advantage of the size and height of a street punk. One of my student's original instructors was only five feet tall, maybe one hundred pounds. She – yes, *she* - used to throw him all the time, and he was five foot ten inches tall and weighed two hundred and ten pounds. She knows how to execute techniques with minimum effort and maximum efficiency.

LWC: All things being equal except for physical strength, who will win in a fight, the muscular strong guy or the non-weight trained fighter?

TD: This is a hypothesis that would probably never happen. Nothing is equal in all other aspects. However, not to evade the question, it would make sense the muscular strong guy would win over the non-weight-trained fighter. But there is always the element of luck that could change this outcome.

LWC: Is it realistic to think that a jujitsu fighter can catch a punch and apply a lock on that arm?

TD: Remember we are talking about training a person in jujitsu for self-defense in the streets. If against an average street fighter I think it is very reasonable to think a trained jujitsu person could catch the arm and apply a lock. However, if it's against another trained fighter, it's not realistic. But again, Lady Luck often plays a big role in a fight.

LWC: What are the weaknesses in jujitsu?

TD: There are none! Just kidding, but think about it: Jujitsu was developed centuries ago and blends many martial arts of war. Samurais in each village or region developed their own hand fighting techniques. They had to learn what to do if they were disarmed. They probably didn't say, "If I kick or punch, it's karate" or "If I execute a throw or use a wristlock technique, that's jujitsu." Their aim was to protect their lord and master by any means possible. Each village kept their arsenal secret. If it were revealed, their village could be attacked and they could have their own methods used against them.

Years ago our jujitsu system was somewhat weak when it came to the striking arts. So Professor Moore insisted that all his jujitsu students train in karate. In fact, to progress past fifth dan in jujitsu, the student had to have a black belt in karate.

Probably the greatest weakness is the length of time and practice required to learn a system, then on to other systems. That's probably why the greatest masters are always pictured as being so old.

LWC: What are some of the other beliefs about jujitsu that simply aren't true?

TD: That question was asked in one of our classes recently. One student said that he thought jujitsu was only about throwing. He has since learned that jujitsu really is a blend of many techniques.

A jujitsu instructor friend of mine says, "Jujitsu is translated to mean 'gentle art' but if it doesn't hurt then it's not jujitsu." I agree: there is nothing gentle about it.

LWC: How would you fight a superior puncher? How would you fight a superior kicker?

TD: We teach street jujitsu with an emphasis on avoiding a fight at all costs. It's not worth your money, watch, or your ring to get hurt. Or for you to hurt someone else. But if you have to defend yourself or someone close to you, ascertain to the best of your ability if the attacker is a puncher or kicker.

Since punchers don't normally use their feet, their weak point is their legs. Go in for leg sweeps or leg takedowns. If the attacker is a kicker, his weak point would probably be his upper body. Move in close so he can't use his legs. Joint lock techniques or upper body throws would probably work well. Most important, don't play their game. Play to your strengths, not theirs.

LWC: Once and for all, how easy would it be to break a limb or even kill an attacker with jujitsu?

TD: If one has the skills, it's very easy to maim or kill. Let's take them one at a time.

Many people have the misconception that we break arms and legs. That's really not true. We dislocate elbows and knees. And we crack ribs. I think it only takes 8 to 12 pounds of pressure to dislocate a joint. Actually, how much pressure to crack a limb is very conjectural. It would depend on how it's supported and the angle and power of the strike or throw. Throwing an untrained person onto concrete might cause several limbs to break. My wife saw a person break his arm in two places during practice on a padded mat. But if you throw a well-trained person on a concrete surface, he might sustain only bruises.

In fact, one of my students fell several feet onto a concrete pier and received only bruises. Another rolled off a motorcycle, tore up his gloves and hobbled away with only a sprained ankle.

The same applies for killing an attacker. In this chapter, we illustrate a couple of techniques that could easily kill. So obviously you must practice with safety in mind. Do things slowly and do them well before trying anything more advanced.

LWC: How important is the environment when using jujitsu for self-defense?

TD: Always be aware of your surroundings, all of your environment. Be aware of your escape routes and items you might use for self-defense. In the demonstrated techniques in this chapter, we took full advantage of the environment: a chair, a wall, and the floor. If you're in the woods, use a tree branch, the actual tree, and the ground. In the city, use a mailbox, telephone pole, or concrete curb.

While these objects are highly effective, always remember that your brain is your best weapon. Use it to get yourself out of trouble.

LWC: Are some styles of jujitsu more street oriented than are others?

TD: There are many schools and types of jujitsu. They range from the very formal, classical ones to the strictly modern street self-defense styles. Some schools practice with real knives instead of the wooden ones that we use. Our system allows our schools a great deal of flexibility. We teach in a safe environment and explain what to do to enhance a technique in the streets. Our founder, Professor Duke Moore, tossed out techniques, changed techniques, and came up with new ones that were more street oriented.

LWC: Are some teachers taking the formality and culture protocols out of jujitsu and making it more street oriented?

TD: As I said, our schools have a great deal of latitude. Each places a different emphasis on culture and technique while trying to balance the needs of the students. There is only so much time available to teach culture and techniques. Even within the San Francisco Bay Area our schools range from the formal to the informal. By formal I mean following the traditional openings. I think we are all very informal as to how we are addressed. As an instructor, I don't insist on being called sensei, professor, master professor, or grandmaster. The students insist on the formal address. Although we maintain the formalities, we don't strictly adhere to only one way of doing things.

We think of ourselves as a modern traditional style. Our techniques are conformed to the needs of our modern times. For example, the samurai had a need to know how to defend themselves from a kneeling position, a position where in their culture they meditated, talked, and so on. In our society, this is not a common position, so it's one that we only address lightly.

The simple but devastating techniques shown here are just a few of Soke Delgman's favorites. Since they are quite dangerous, he says to practice them slowly and maintain control at all times. He says, "No matter how many pictures you look at, there is no substitute for a qualified instructor. One must learn the *feel* of the technique and practice on different body types to become proficient. Remember, not all techniques work on all people all of the time. That is why a qualified instructor is needed to help you find variations that apply specifically to you."

Finger dislocation defense against a grab attack while seated

You're sitting in a restaurant, a park, or a bar, when an attacker lunges for you. Twist your body aside as you reach for his closest hand. In this case your left hand to his right.

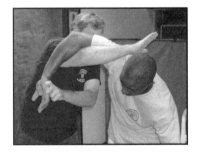

Wrap your pinky and ring finger around the attacker's pinky, with your index and middle finger at the meaty part of the hand. Pull to stretch the pinky while wrapping your thumb around the attacker's hand or wrist.

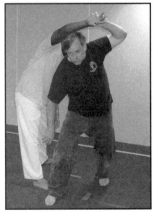

Stand up quickly and dip under the attacker's arm while applying intense pressure to his finger.

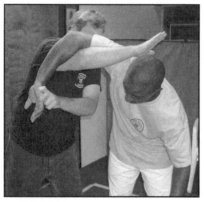

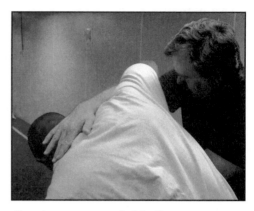

As you continue to stretch his pinky painfully across his other fingers, reach under his arm and grab the back of his head.

Continue to stretch his finger as you push his head to drive him through an open door, into a wall, or over a table.

Smash with chair defense against a grab while seated

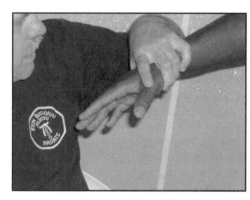

You're sitting peacefully when you're attacked. Grab the attacker's right hand with your left. Your fingers will encircle his wrist at the base of his thumb as your thumb presses into the back of his hand just below the knuckles.

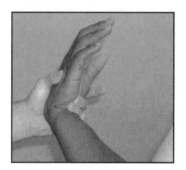

Twist his hand so that his palm faces him.

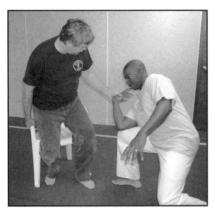

Stand and grab the chair behind you as you twist until he drops to one knee. Apply pressure to his hand by pulling towards your body with your fingers while simultaneously pushing towards the attacker with your thumb. Continue applying pressure by pulling with your fingers and pushing with your thumb. Twist to your left while pulling your arm down to your left side.

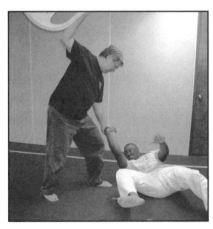

Keep twisting until he falls to the floor. Grab a chair and smash him with it.

Throw attacker onto chair defense against an attack while seated

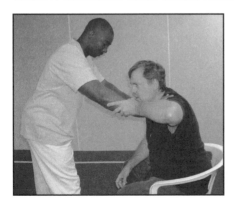

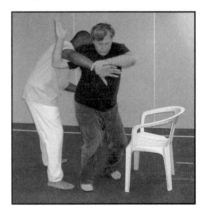

An attacker moves to choke you. Grab his left upper forearm. Step forward with your right foot while turning it and your body to face the chair.

Your right hand goes under the attacker's right biceps and then shoots upward. Your left hand slides down his arm to his wrist.

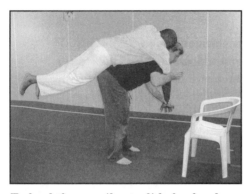

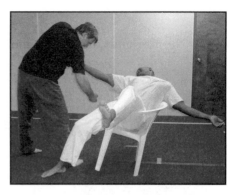

To load the assailant, slide back, place your feet together, and bend your knees. The throw occurs when you pull with your left hand and thrust with your right as you bend forward.

Throw the assailant over your right shoulder and onto a chair.

Note: Throwing your training partner onto a chair is likely to cause injury. To be safe, stop practicing at the previous step.

Throw attacker into a wall from a standing attack

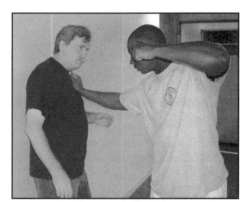

You're standing against a wall and an attacker grabs your shirt, pushes you back and starts to punch you.

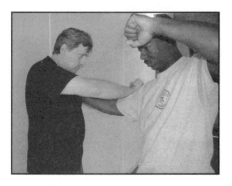

As you're pushed back, quickly place your right wrist palm down across the attacker's right arm and clasp hands with your left. Depending on how quickly the situation unfolds, you might have to block the punch first.

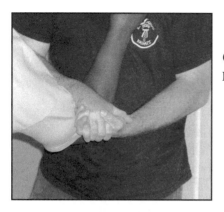

Close-up, reverse view of the previous step.

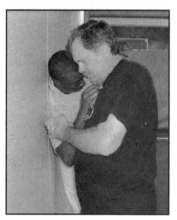

To bring the attacker's elbow into your body, move your left hand downward while rotating the back of your right hand toward the attacker. Step toward the wall with your right leg to drive him into it.

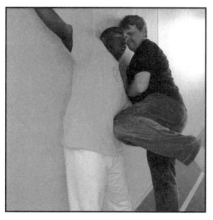

Finish him with a knee slam.

Note: As mentioned throughout this book, be careful in your training and be justified to use the severe level of force demonstrated in these photos.

Soke **Tim Delgman**'s introduction to the martial arts was through his uncle, Art Buckley, in 1970 at the age of 10. In the decades since Tim has earned a 9th-degree black belt in jujitsu, a 1st-degree black belt in Wado Ki Kai karate, a 1st-degree black belt in judo, an honorary 6th-degree black belt in Miyami Ryu jujitsu, and in 2004, he became the soke, the inheritor of the Zen Budo Kai system of aiki jujitsu.

Tim Delgman is a quiet, well-informed man in a variety of areas, to include bird watching, model train collecting, camping, photography, and travel. Tim's wife Rosa and son Joseph are martial arts practitioners making it a family affair.

As is the case with many veteran martial artists, Tim appears to be a mild mannered person, a teacher whose philosophy is to avoid street violence, but get him on the mat...

The Zen Budo Kai main dojo is in San Francisco, California. Although they do very little advertising, students find them by word of mouth or through the internet at www.zenbudokai.com. Besides teaching at the main San Francisco school, Soke Delgman also teaches in Pleasant Hill and routinely assists Irving Lee at his school in Walnut Creek and Doug Haight at his in Orinda.

Many thanks to Purtis E. Marks for his work as my opponent, and to Rosa Maria Delgman and Irving Lee for their fine work behind the camera.

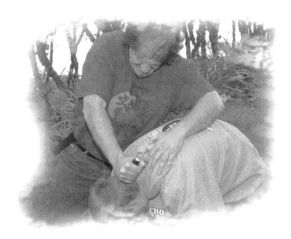

SECTION FIVE
WEAPONS

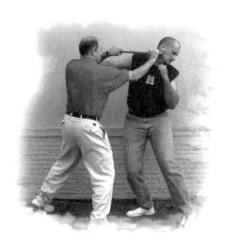

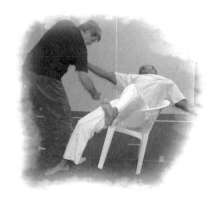

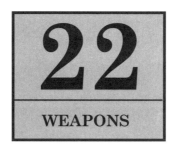

11 Ways to Use an Impact Tool for Self-Defense

By Dan Anderson

You wouldn't think a chapter on how to use an impact tool *against* an attacker would be in this book. It would seem that it would be more about how to defend against an attacker wielding one. Well, there are many volumes covering that subject but precious little covering the approach that I'm taking here.

An impact tool is probably man's oldest weapon. Far before the forging of steel was the easy availability of a stick. It was easy to find, easy to pick up, and definitely easy to hit someone with. It was one of the first equalizers. Today, there are many different kinds of impact tools, ranging from crowbars to bottles, ASP batons to tightly rolled magazines, and hammers to car antennas. They all have one thing in common: you pick up the tool and swing it. Here are some tips to do it well.

The impact art of arnis

Many martial arts styles use a stick of some kind as a fighting tool. I practice the Filipino art of arnis, which is applicable to any impact tool. The arnis training I have had forms the basis of this chapter.

Note: I demonstrate the following techniques using a stick. Anytime I write the word "stick" keep in mind that I actually mean impact tool. A tightly rolled magazine will do nearly the same damage as a hardwood stick, and you have access to a magazine more often than you do a stick.

You wouldn't think that anyone would attack somebody who was armed with a stick or any other kind of weapon. It seems that the attacker would think that the defender, the one armed, would have an advantage. However, a key point about people who attack others is that they always feel that they have the advantage, whether they do or not. Also, just because a person picks up a weapon doesn't mean that he actually has faith in his ability to use it. Hence this chapter.

Stance

If you have the time to get into some kind of preparatory position, count yourself one of the lucky ones. A *sudden attack* does not leave much time to get prepared. Preparation is a state of mind along with some common sense. You can use any kind of ready position if you know you have the need to use your weapon. I prefer the two pictured here.

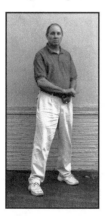

The hidden position. I have the stick tucked under my arm, concealed, but ready for a fast forward strike or block.

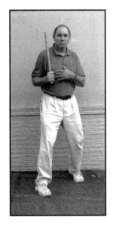

The guard position. This lets your opponent know that you mean business. The stick is vertical, ready to strike or deflect.

If you're new to any kind of stick defense, know that it is best to keep your actions extremely simple. Your blocks and strikes need to be short, fast, and powerful. The acronym KISS (keep it simple, stupid) is key, as attacks are often fast and sudden. Reliance on fancy or intricate actions is only for the incredibly well-trained fighter, and even they will tell you to keep it simple.

Examples of impact tool defense

Two-handed grip:

Defense against a punch

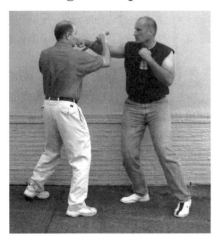

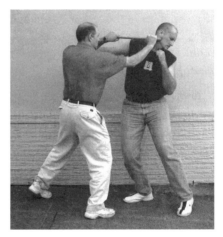

As your attacker swings, use a two-handed grip to move your stick into the way of his strike. He helps provide the impact on his arm. Hey, he hit at you. He might as well provide some of the pain.

From the block, immediately ram your stick straight into the side of his jaw or cheekbone.

On commitment

You can't begin a defense and then back off hoping that your assailant will take pity on you and go away. When you cross that line and take any kind of defensive or counter-offensive action, you're committed for the duration. You need to follow all of your defenses with a counter strike or a series of counter strikes to keep your attacker from continuing his aggression. I know this is preaching to the choir, but you would be surprised at how many people balk at the thought of hitting an attacker.

Defense against a kick

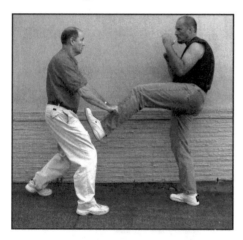

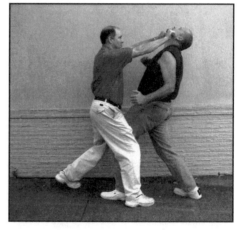

Jam the stick downward into your attacker's shin as he kicks.

From this point, bring your stick straight up into his face. You're using the rebound off his shin as impetus for your strike. It doesn't matter if you hit him in the nose, chin or throat. Your objective is to defend yourself and get out of there.

One-handed grip:

Defense against an aggressive reach or punch

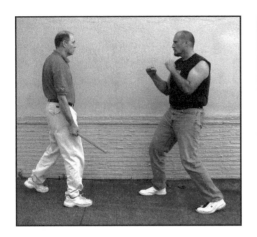 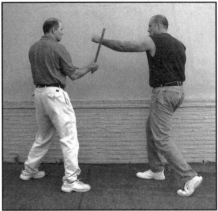

Just as your attacker hits or reaches at you, fire the stick sharply from its down position into the attacking limb.

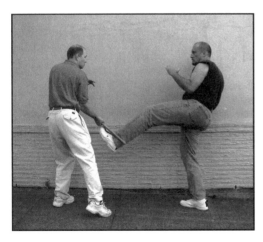

It doesn't matter whether you rap his arm (against a punch) or his shin (against a kick); sharp impact with the stick helps your defense. If you have an ASP baton, a nightstick, or a big flashlight, that sharp impact will give your attacker pause. Again, once you have done this you probably will need to hit two or three more times to ensure that you stop him long enough for you make a clean get away.

Defense against a combination attack

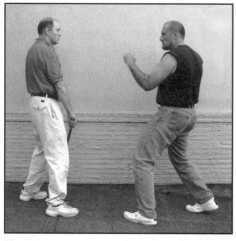
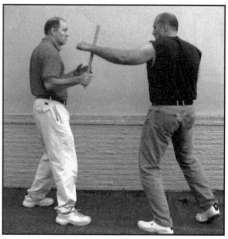

You can use your stick to deliver a combination parry/strike to your opponent's punch or reach. He jabs, and you meet it meet with your stick.

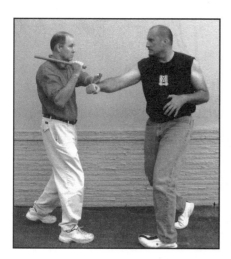
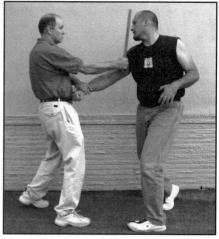

Your hand parries his follow-up punch.

Counter with a strike to his head with your stick.

This action takes a bit of training to pull off well. It's not because it's complex but because of the timing. It's a good one to train because there is no rule that an attacker has only one try at one punch and then he goes home. If he fires at you once, there is no reason to believe he won't fire on you again. Therefore, it's beneficial to work against multiple attacks. You can use any of the examples in this chapter and then compound them to create training scenarios.

Defense against a stick grab

This will be a problem only if you make a big production out of it. Years ago, my teacher, Professor Remy Presas, told me not to get hypnotized by the stick. As years went by, I noticed that whenever I grabbed someone's stick, the first thing the person did was to make a big effort of getting it back. He was so wrapped up in the fact that he "lost" a weapon that he forgot he had three others: another hand and two feet.

When your opponent grabs your stick

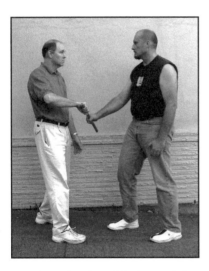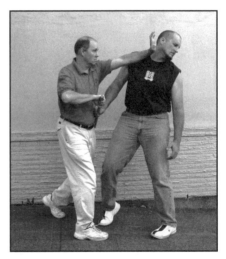

You just fire into his face with your other hand. This is not flashy nor is it very exciting. Your opponent is somewhat "hypnotized by your stick." He has placed his attention on it or he would not have grabbed it in the first place. He either wants it or wants to immobilize it. Great! Hit him – fast and hard.

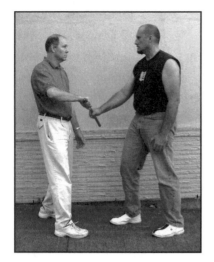
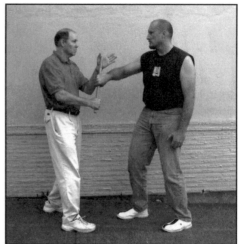

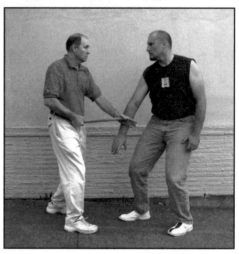

Go for a simple release. Up-end your stick with your opposite hand and then push it downward. This affects a release and then you can follow up with a hit. When you up-end your stick, you draw your grab-hand back to your side to control his arm and to set up your other hand to push. You coordinate your downward push of the arm to fire your stick upward into his face for your counter strike. This takes more physical and mental coordination to pull off than does simply smacking your attacker. When in doubt, keep it simple.

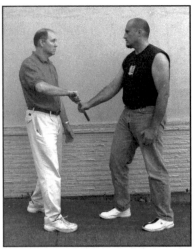
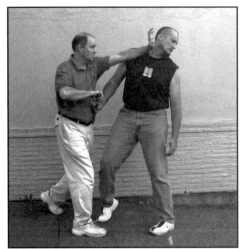
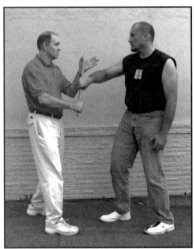
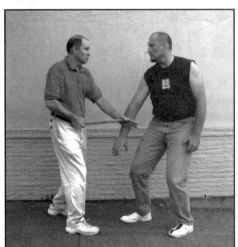

You can also hit first as he grips the stick, then release it as just shown and hit again. When you look at the illustration photos you will see that you can interchange the actions somewhat.

Distraction

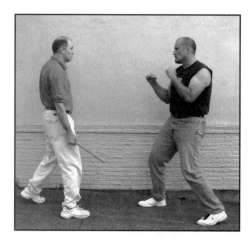 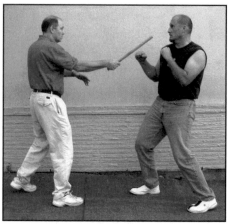

Inserting a distraction is often overlooked as an effective set up. Flick the tip of your stick straight up towards your attacker's face. A person's usual reaction is to brush it aside, flinch, pull away, or whatever.

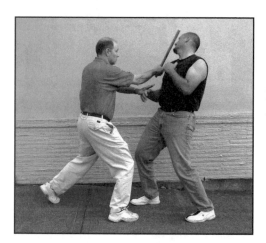

It doesn't matter because from there you will go on the attack.

Hit and run

This action is another simple overlooked concept. Many people believe that once you begin to defend yourself, you need to fight to the finish. Well, you do need to be *willing* to fight to the finish if that is what it is going to take, but quite often a hit and run tactic is all that's needed.

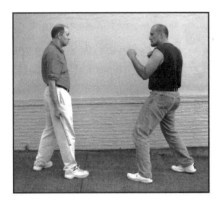

You're facing a menacing threat.

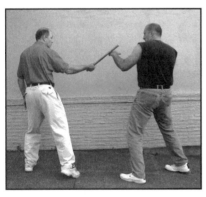

Use your stick to hit hard whatever target is the closest.

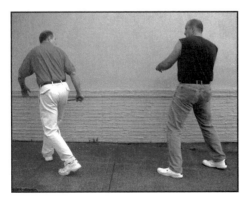

Upon impact, turn, and run. You hit and you split! You can gain some good distance on you assailant before he begins to attack you again...if he does.

Remember, self-defense is not a Jackie Chan movie. You don't have the luxury of having a script that says you are the winner and besides, how often do you have access to a ladder and bench like Jackie does, anyway?

Striking With Power

It doesn't mean anything if you have an impact tool in your hand but you don't put any "juice" behind it. I was at a gas station one night and watched as a female police officer tried to get a suspected drug dealer out of his car. The threat of a gun pointed at him did no good; he just stayed inside. So she pulled out her collapsible baton and began beating on the passenger window, shattering it in seconds. She went to the other side of the car and did the same to the driver's-side window.

The guy did come out of his car but then he went immediately to his trunk! The officer swung her baton at his head but her body action checked the power of her swing, that is, she unconsciously pulled her swing. Instead of hammering this guy like she did on his side windows, she just bonked him. His reaction? He said "Ow!"

Then he went about rummaging through his trunk. She fired on him again. He raised his arm. She pulled her body back a second time, and again he uttered an "Ow." Then he took off in a sprint and got away.

I sat there amazed. She had two opportunities to drop this guy colder than a sack of fish and she checked her swing every time. She was missing two things – intention and body mechanics. Let's take up the mechanics first.

Mechanics of power striking

Nearly everyone knows how to hit a ball, whether it is a baseball or a tennis ball. The mechanics are the same. You swing into the pitch. It is the same with any kind of strike with an impact tool. You turn into it so that you can get your body behind it. The police officer turned *away* while hitting forward, thus killing the power of her strike.

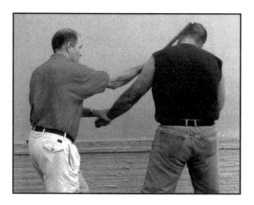 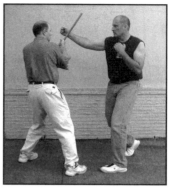

If you look at the photos for the forehand strikes, you'll notice that I turn into the strike; I get my weight into it, just not the power of my arm.

In practice you will stop your *partner* if you hit him with an arm-based strike. He is a partner, not an enemy. But in the heat of an attack, your enemy might just walk through anything delivered with less than full power. A good way to tell if you have power in a strike is to hit the heavy bag with a stick. What does your body tell you? Did it feel solid? Did you only feel it in your arm? Did it feel like your whole body connected?

Intention

The police officer lacked intent, too. Even if she had had good body mechanics, she might not have had any effect due to lack of intention.

This brings up an interesting point regarding the use of any kind of weapon. Jaye Spiro is a well-known self-defense teacher. Once when she was at my school for a seminar, she said that she didn't recommend women carrying a knife unless they had the *emotional content* to use it. This is a very important point.

Are you willing to hit someone with an impact tool with intent? If not, you have no business carrying one. If you do carry one be willing to use it and, put your body into it. Whether you decide to train in an art that specializes in impact tools or if you just pick up a few tips from this chapter, learn it and learn it well. It could save your life.

Here is an anecdote that illustrates what I mean by intention. I was driving home from work a number of years ago when I saw a couple of guys fighting in the street. One man held the other in a headlock and was beating him in the face. My first thought was, "This looks bad." I was thinking about appearance rather than the severity of the situation. I decided to handle it.

It was during rush hour so I had to wait for traffic to clear to make a left turn so that I could park my car. A few more minutes passed before I could make it across the street. When I approached these two, they were squared off at each other. As I walked up to them I was thinking, "This is really stupid. What have I gotten myself into? They could easily turn on me."

As I approached, I veered slightly toward the guy to my right thinking that if they did start in on me, I had a clear shot at him; I was going to drop him fast if need be.

I stopped out of range of the two guys, and said loud and clear, "Hi!"

They turned around and walked off.

I couldn't believe it. The trouble that I had mentally prepared for didn't happen. When I examined the incident later, I found an answer to what had happened. My intention was to stop the fight, even if it turned on me.

That intention came through in a single word: "Hi!" That's what I'm talking about.

The use of an impact tool relies on three key points:

- Simple actions are the best

- Learn how to hit *hard* with the tool

- Be *willing* to hit hard with the tool

Train hard.

*D*an **Anderson** began studying karate with me in November of 1966 when I was teaching a style called kongsu, a Korean form of Shotokan karate. I was teaching beginning, intermediate and advanced classes then and though Dan was only 14 years old when he started, I immediately recognized that there was something special about him. His ability to instantly grasp techniques and concepts was amazing. Within a couple of months he asked if he could attend the intermediate class, and I said yes. Three or four months after that, he asked if he could slip into the advanced class. I allowed that, too. There was no holding this kid back

A year and half later I went into the Army for three years and Dan continued to study under my instructor, Bruce Terrill. When I got out of the service, Dan was a black belt and well on his way to making a huge name for himself on the tournament circuit.

I'd like to take credit for Dan's accomplishments but all I did was get him started. His success comes from an inquisitive mind, hard training, and his relationships with some of the best in the martial arts since the 1960s.

Here is a little of what he has accomplished during his long martial arts career.
• Promoted to 1st-degree black belt in January of 1970
• Founded American Freestyle Karate, one of the first styles of American kazate.
• Was the only competitor in America to be rated in both Black Belt and Karate Illustrated magazine as a Top Ten fighter of the year.
• Won over 70 Grand Championship titles.
• Rated in the Top Five Referees in the United States.
• Author of 10 books on karate and Modern Arnis.
• Double Gold Medalist in the 1990 Seattle Goodwill Games Karate competition (WUKO rules).
• Promoted to 6th-degree black belt in Modern Arnis on On June 28, 1992 by Grand Master Remy A. Presas. Awarded Senior Master status in 1995.
• Promoted to 7th-degree black belt in by the American Teachers Association of the Martial Arts on April 16, 1996.
• Granted permission by Grand Master Remy A. Presas to establish his own branch of Modern Arnis.

• Received the Founder Of The Year award in 2002 by the World Head Of Family Sokeship Council for the formation of the MA-80 style of Modern Arnis.

• Came out of retirement in 2002 to win the 50- to 54-years-of-age division of the Funakoshi Shotokan Karate Association 4th World Championships.

• Received recognition in 2003 for founding MA-80 Modern Arnis and an 8th-degree black belt from Professor Wally Jay, Bong Jornales, Dr. Maung Gyi and Gat Puno Abon Baet.

See more about Dan Anderson and check out his books, DVDs and film clips on his website at www.danandersonkarate.com.

A big thanks to Tom Corsin for posing as the attacker and to Justin Mangum for the great photos.

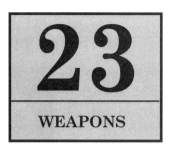

12 Ways to Fight With a Mini Flashlight

By Loren W. Christensen

I first discovered the effectiveness of a flashlight when I served as a patrolman with the U.S. Army's Military Police Unit in Saigon. I acquired a 15-inch long unit that had the most intense light beam I'd ever seen. I don't recall where I got it or any details as to its construction, but I do remember the intensity of that light. I wouldn't be surprised if it could have been seen from space.

I worked nights then with a couple other MPs. I would shine that laser-like beam into alleyways, onto second-story balconies, and up on rooftops, and watch as people in hiding - Vietnamese violating curfew, AWOL American GIs, drunks, dopers, prostitutes, and every other type of night creature – slithered away from the intense illumination and disappear to places even the light couldn't reach. It was at once fun and a little sobering to realize how many eyes were on us, at least until I zapped them with my super-killer light beam.

A bit of technical stuff

My flashlight then was quite large, but today there are mini versions, 5-inches in length that emit the same intense light and, with some models, light many times greater. Now, I'm not going to go into the specifics of candlepower, LEDs, and all kinds of technical data that I would be lying if I said I understood or even cared about. I'm not technically minded and I'm okay with that (hey, I've survived this long without all that stuff in my head). However, the interested reader can research easily enough on the internet and by studying the specs provided by the many manufacturers of these flashlights. Did you know that there are even internet forums where people sit around and talk about flashlights? Sheesh!

For our purposes, all you need is a small light that you can clench in your fist and slip into your back pocket without its weight pulling your trousers down. Make sure it's constructed with a solid alloy that can withstand a hard whack to an assailant's skull. Your light should also have a tailcap switch that allows you to activate the beam by a press of your thumb and to shut off the light when you move your thumb away.

For self-defense, a sudden, thumb-activated light beam in a bully's eyes will make him jerk his head away and curse you. That tactic always worked well for me in police work, even with a cheap-o flashlight. But when the same tactic is used with today's super-duper mini-light beams, even a choirboy would scrunch his eyes shut and curse your mother's birth. One of my students brought one to class one day, a model that cost him serious money, and flipped it on in my face. Even in the well-lit room, the beam was excruciating. If it had been a self-defense situation, he could have easily followed with a quick kick to the groin.

While the tailcap switch is recommended, if you can find a model that has a quick on-and-off switch on the barrel of the flashlight that you can activate just as easily under stress, that will serve your purpose, too. Remember, your small motor skills are the first to go in an adrenaline-pumping situation.

How to carry

Cops will talk for hours about the many ways to carry their firearms. But we're talking about a flashlight here so let's not get carried away. Here are some simple suggestions.

- **In your home:** Place it anywhere it's easily accessible, which means not in the bottom of your kitchen junk drawer or out in the garage. It's small, so you can put it behind that vase on the shelf by the door, on top of the refrigerator, or on your nightstand. Keep it in one place so you know exactly where it is should you lose electricity or you hear a bump in the night.

- **In your car**: If you put it in your glove box it will likely work its way to the bottom of all the junk you stuff in there. A better place might be in the ashtray, a change holder, the door panel, or the coffee holder. Put it wherever you have quick access should you break down at night or a road-rager comes stomping up to your door.

- **On your person**: Where you carry your mini light depends on your preference, lifestyle, and the situation. If your lifestyle is routine, carry it in your pocket. If your day takes you to potentially rough parts of town, you might want to carry it on your pants belt in its own little holster, of which there are many variations. If you're in a high-risk situation, such as walking on a dark sidewalk, crossing a poorly lit parking lot, or checking the outside of your house for that strange bump you heard, you might want to carry it at the ready in your hand.

Let's look at a simple way to strike with the mini flashlight. With the basic technique I suggest here and the striking set I offer as a foundation for thinking about directions of force, the creative reader can devise dozens of techniques. In the end, it's all about simplicity and gross motor movement.

Hammer fist

Consider the hammer fist, sometimes called bottom fist. You use the hammer fist when you pound the heel of your fist on a table in anger, on your steering wheel in a moment of road rage, or at a martial arts demonstration when you smash that huge block of ice that wasn't doing anything to you. By whatever name, it's a powerful hand strike, arguably the most powerful in the kick/punch arts. It's not used as much as other hand strikes because an opponent can easily see it coming, but when it does land it has a high potential to cause pain and destruction to collar bones, necks, and giant ice cubes.

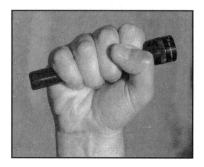

Here is a way to make the technique even nastier: Hold a small pipe in your fist, one that is really a flashlight.

Be justified to hit

Yes the tiny flashlight is almost toy-like and they can be purchased in pretty blues, reds and yellows, but they are nonetheless a metal rod, and that is exactly how the police and the court will see them should you use yours in a fight that isn't justified.

As you try to convince the judge in a squeaky little baby voice, "It's just a whittle, teenie-tiny light I use to find my keys at night," the prosecution, in a deep, rumbling voice will argue, "The defendant used an iron rod to smash this poor, weak man in his head as he begged for food for his starving baby." Then the prosecution will hand the iron-hard flashlight to the jury and ask each one to tap it against their forehead and imagine it hitting them many times harder. (Yes, things do get this twisted around in court.)

As I've noted throughout this book, any time you use force against another person you must be justified. It's arguably even more critical when you use a weapon, and a "teenie-tiny light" is a weapon when it's used to slam against a head. Use only that force needed to stop the threat or clear a path for you to escape. Then run away.

While you don't benefit from centrifugal force as you do when you swing a stick, pole, or a steel ball with spikes protruding from the end of a chain, you will benefit from an inch or two of circular metal jutting out one or both sides of your tightly clenched, enhanced fist. You can strike with either end.

Fist

When you squeeze a small, cylindrical tube that is a flashlight within your clenched hand, your fist instantly becomes tight and hard. There is less give to the fingers on impact and people struck say that they can definitely feel the difference. Clenching the mini-light enhances straight-line punches, hooks and backfists. Unlike with the hammer fist, however, it's only the fist that makes impact, not the hard, protruding flashlight.

Use the enhanced straight punch to slam an assailant with a single blow to his upper chest plate, solar plexus, or ribs. In a combination, use a fast enhanced straight punch to first drill your assailant in the body to distract him from seeing you chamber your arm for the more visually obvious, but harder hitting hammer fist.

Hammer fist striking set

The following striking set is more about directions of force and striking at different levels than it is about hitting specific targets. However, I've listed body parts here so you have a target to strike when you're first learning to hit with the mini-light or when you want to warm-up with a partner.

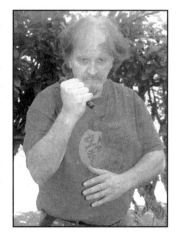

In this on-guard position (right), the weapon is in your strong hand with the same leg forward to give you maximum reach, though you can place your other leg forward if that is more comfortable.

From here you can easily deliver a continuous series of strikes to the following 11 targets. For example, strike downward to the top of the head, retract the weapon and strike his left temple. Retract and strike his other temple. Continue in this fashion down your opponent's body until you have delivered an uppercut with the light into your opponent's groin. Here is the set:

1. Strike top of head
2. Strike left temple
3. Strike right temple
4. Strike left neck
5. Strike right neck
6. Strike right ribs
7. Strike left ribs
8. Strike solar plexus
9. Uppercut strike to the groin
10. Strike behind you to hit groin
11. Jab over your shoulder behind you to hit the face

Once you're comfortable with this striking set, which shouldn't take you longer than one or two workouts, you're ready to begin experimenting with different self-defense scenarios. You will immediately see that there is a whole smorgasbord of targets available to you when you think in terms of angles, or directions of force. While the places to hit will vary, depending on a host of variables in a fight, the directions of force remain constant, whether you're standing, kneeling, lying down, or hanging upside down for some odd reason. Here are three examples from the set:

Number 1: strike downward In the set, you just strike the top of the head, but there are many more targets available when you think in terms of striking downward. The flashlight rule is this: Whatever is available, hit it.

Targets

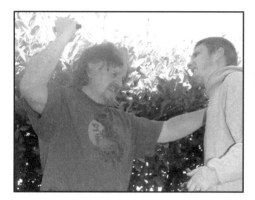

From a downward strike, hit:

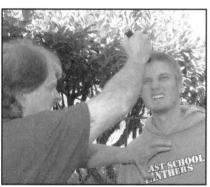

Top of head

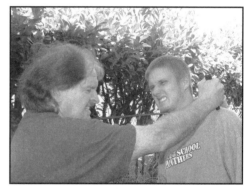

Top of shoulder

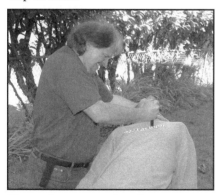

Face, chest or groin when
the assailant is bent over backwards

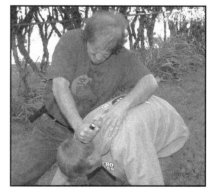

Back of head, back of neck or spine
when the assailant is bent forwards

407

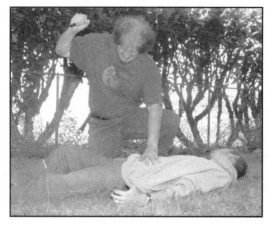 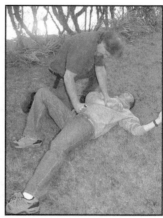

Face, neck, chest, arms, hands, groin, or legs when the assailant is lying face up

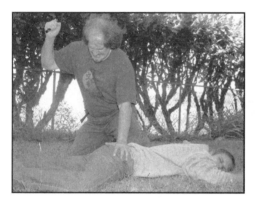 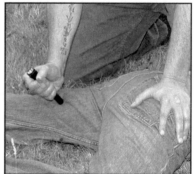

Head, neck, spine, arms, hands, or legs when the assailant is lying face down

Number 2, strike from your left Hit whatever is available when the path is open from your left to right.

Targets

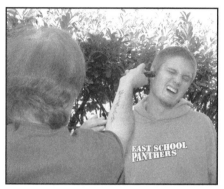

Right temple when you and the assailant are standing (notice the inverted hand position option)

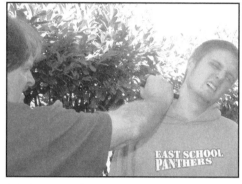

Right side of neck when you and the assailant are standing

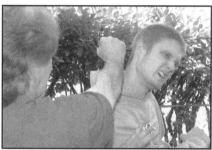

Face or back of head when you're perpendicular to the assailant

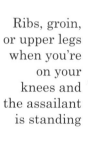 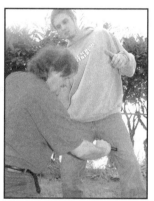

Ribs, groin, or upper legs when you're on your knees and the assailant is standing

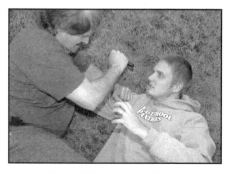 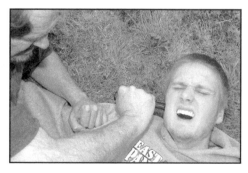

Any vulnerable target when you and the assailant are both on the ground.

Number 9, upward strike   Hit whatever is available when there is an upward path open.

Targets

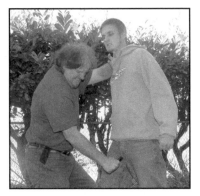

Groin when you and the assailant are standing.

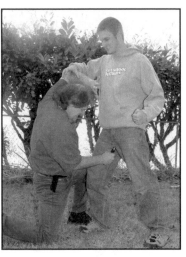

Groin when you're kneeling and the assailant is standing.

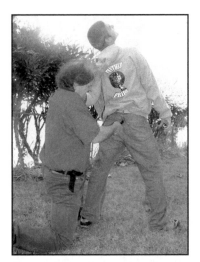

Coccyx bone (upper butt) when you and the assailant are standing and he is facing away.

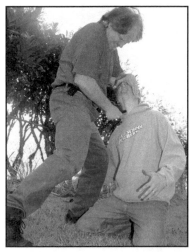

Throat when the assailant is kneeling and you're standing.

Number 10, backward and upward strike Hit whatever is available when there is a backward and upward path open.

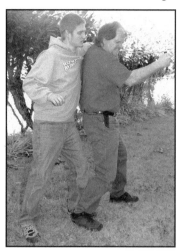

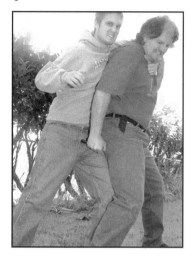

The set up for both the groin and the head targets.

Hit the groin when attacked and the from behind.

Number 11, hit over your shoulder and behind you Hit when there is a pathway available to a target over your shoulder and behind you.

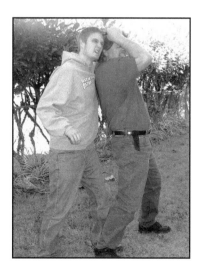

Target: Face when attacked from behind.

I could go through the entire striking set this way but you get the idea. Just know that the 11-count striking set is a device to introduce angles and directions of force. You can use any angle of attack whenever and wherever you have a target available.

What about the light?

As mentioned earlier, it's preferred that your light have a tailcap switch that you can activate for one or two disorientating seconds, at which time you can punch, kick or smash the threat with your flashlight. While it would seem that this would be most effective during the hours of darkness, some lights are so intense they make an assailant blink and look away even on a sunny day. Ideally, however, your situation will occur during the hours of darkness.

Phil Elmore, author of *Flashlight Fighting*, published by Paladin Press, said this about the power of light. "When you are facing an assailant in low-light conditions, your ability to suddenly flood his pupils with bright light gives you a very real physical advantage. There are no guarantees that you will blind him or sufficiently discourage him with light alone, but most people find the sudden transition from night lighting to, say, 60 lumens of Xenon-bulb torch light to be physically disabling for at least a fraction of a second. Most people instinctively flinch away from such bright light. Many will blink repeatedly while reflexively bringing their hands up in front of their faces."

That's when you hit them.

Pressing and rubbing

You can also use either end of your light to press or rub vulnerable targets. These techniques hurt unless the recipient is under the influence of drugs, alcohol, rage, or is mentally ill, conditions that cause some people to be impervious to pain. Therefore, don't count on these techniques to be the end all, but rather a potentially painful supplement to a grappling technique you're already applying.

Targets to rub and press

Head area, especially the face	Neck, especially the front
Chest plate	Pectorals
Biceps	Triceps
Back of hands	Either side of wrist
Ribs	Groin
Inner thigh	Inside knee
Shin	Calf

Here are three examples to double the pain.

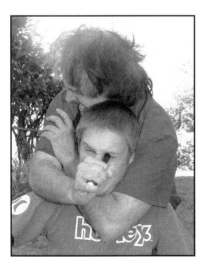

Apply a carotid sleeper by compressing the artery with your left biceps on the left side of the assailant's neck and with your forearm on the right side. The biceps of your right arm pulls your left forearm in tight against the neck as you press the end of the flashlight into his eye.

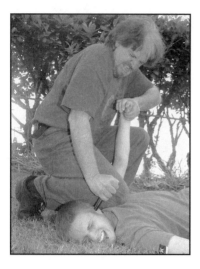

Assume any arm control technique you like while your opponent is lying on his stomach. In this case, I'm jamming his wrist, hyperextending his elbow joint, stretching and jamming his shoulder joint. If needed, I can add even more pain by pressing the flashlight into his ear canal.

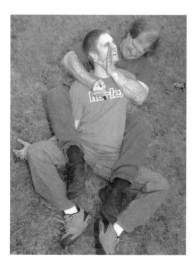

You have been thrashing about on the ground with your attacker and have maneuvered him into a position where you can completely control his arms and have fair control over his lower half. Since my opponent is quite strong, he begins to force his upper body forward as if to escape. To keep him in place, I press the end of the metal mini-light into his chest plate and rub it back and forth forcefully a few inches in each direction. Most people have very little meat there, which makes them quite vulnerable to this technique.

Easy (and fun) training: attack the innocent

You're in a line at the movie theater, sitting in a restaurant, or on the subway. It doesn't matter where you are as long as there are people around you. They are innocent people; not a troublemaker among them. Still, you're going to whack them with your steel pipe-like flashlight. See that guy there? Strike him in the face. That teenager over in the corner? Smack his groin. That stockbroker-looking man? Whack his spine.

Okay, you're not really going to hit these nice people but you are in your mind. It's mental imagery practice, visualization. You see the target, you devise the angle of attack given where it is, and you mentally attack it.

Let's say you're sitting down in a subway car. Imagine you have your flashlight in your right hand, an inch protruding out of each side of your fist. You're going to mentally hit that guy holding onto the pole and daydreaming. But where? From where?

Say you're holding the light in your fist on your right thigh. Say the daydreamer is two feet from you. What targets are most available? Groin? Inner thigh? Outer thigh? Knee cap? The back of his hand that is gripping the pole? All good ones.

See yourself lash your hand out in what is probably a Number 7 strike, and slam the end of that that steel tube into the nerve on the outside of his upper thigh. Excellent. Do it five more times before he moves.

The next time you're on the subway, your target is sitting and you're standing. You're going to hit him with a Number 1, right on top of his head. Wait until he looks away...now!

See how it works? The more you do it the more you see the targets and understand the angles of attack.

Just don't do it for real.

Loren W. Christensen's biography appears in the "About the Author" page at the back of the book.

Thanks to Jace Widmer for posing with me and to Lisa Christensen for her excellent photography.

Train hard and be safe.
                    Loren W. Christensen

Om Mani Padme Hum

About the author

Loren W. Christensen began his law enforcement career in 1967 as a military policeman in the army and then joined the Portland (Oregon) Police Bureau in 1972, retiring in 1997. During his years on the PPB, he worked street patrol, gang intelligence, dignitary protection, defensive tactics instructor, and riot control.

As a free-lance writer, Loren has authored 34 published books on a variety of subjects, dozens of magazine articles, and edited a newspaper for nearly eight years. He recently coauthored "The evolution of weaponry" with Lt. Col. Dave Grossman for the Encyclopedia of Violence, Peace and Conflict published by Academic Press.

Loren began training in the martial arts in 1965 and continues to this day. He has written over 20 books on the subject and has starred in six instructional DVDs. He has earned a total of 10 black belts, a 7th dan in karate, a 2nd dan in jujitsu, and a 1st dan in arnis.

Loren now writes full time and teaches martial arts to private students and a small group of regulars.

To contact Loren, visit his website LWC Books at www.lwcbooks.com.

NOTES

NOTES

<u>NOTES</u>

NOTES

Index

BOOKS FROM YMAA

6 HEALING MOVEMENTS
101 REFLECTIONS ON TAI CHI CHUAN
108 INSIGHTS INTO TAI CHI CHUAN
ADVANCING IN TAE KWON DO
ANALYSIS OF SHAOLIN CHIN NA 2ND ED
ANCIENT CHINESE WEAPONS
ART OF HOJO UNDO
ARTHRITIS RELIEF, 3RD ED.
BACK PAIN RELIEF, 2ND ED.
BAGUAZHANG, 2ND ED.
CARDIO KICKBOXING ELITE
CHIN NA IN GROUND FIGHTING
CHINESE FAST WRESTLING
CHINESE FITNESS
CHINESE TUI NA MASSAGE
CHOJUN
COMPREHENSIVE APPLICATIONS OF SHAOLIN CHIN NA
CONFLICT COMMUNICATION
CROCODILE AND THE CRANE: A NOVEL
CUTTING SEASON: A XENON PEARL MARTIAL ARTS THRILLER
DEFENSIVE TACTICS
DESHI: A CONNOR BURKE MARTIAL ARTS THRILLER
DIRTY GROUND
DR. WU'S HEAD MASSAGE
DUKKHA HUNGRY GHOSTS
DUKKHA REVERB
DUKKHA, THE SUFFERING: AN EYE FOR AN EYE
DUKKHA UNLOADED
ENZAN: THE FAR MOUNTAIN, A CONNOR BURKE MARTIAL ARTS THRILLER
ESSENCE OF SHAOLIN WHITE CRANE
EXPLORING TAI CHI
FACING VIOLENCE
FIGHT BACK
FIGHT LIKE A PHYSICIST
THE FIGHTER'S BODY
FIGHTER'S FACT BOOK
FIGHTER'S FACT BOOK 2
FIGHTING THE PAIN RESISTANT ATTACKER
FIRST DEFENSE
FORCE DECISIONS: A CITIZENS GUIDE
FOX BORROWS THE TIGER'S AWE
INSIDE TAI CHI
KAGE: THE SHADOW, A CONNOR BURKE MARTIAL ARTS THRILLER
KATA AND THE TRANSMISSION OF KNOWLEDGE
KRAV MAGA PROFESSIONAL TACTICS
KRAV MAGA WEAPON DEFENSES
LITTLE BLACK BOOK OF VIOLENCE
LIUHEBAFA FIVE CHARACTER SECRETS
MARTIAL ARTS ATHLETE
MARTIAL ARTS INSTRUCTION
MARTIAL WAY AND ITS VIRTUES
MASK OF THE KING
MEDITATIONS ON VIOLENCE
MIND/BODY FITNESS
THE MIND INSIDE TAI CHI
THE MIND INSIDE YANG STYLE TAI CHI CHUAN
MUGAI RYU
NATURAL HEALING WITH QIGONG
NORTHERN SHAOLIN SWORD, 2ND ED.
OKINAWA'S COMPLETE KARATE SYSTEM: ISSHIN RYU
POWER BODY
PRINCIPLES OF TRADITIONAL CHINESE MEDICINE
QIGONG FOR HEALTH & MARTIAL ARTS 2ND ED.

QIGONG FOR LIVING
QIGONG FOR TREATING COMMON AILMENTS
QIGONG MASSAGE
QIGONG MEDITATION: EMBRYONIC BREATHING
QIGONG MEDITATION: SMALL CIRCULATION
QIGONG, THE SECRET OF YOUTH: DA MO'S CLASSICS
QUIET TEACHER: A XENON PEARL MARTIAL ARTS THRILLER
RAVEN'S WARRIOR
REDEMPTION
ROOT OF CHINESE QIGONG, 2ND ED.
SCALING FORCE
SENSEI: A CONNOR BURKE MARTIAL ARTS THRILLER
SHIHAN TE: THE BUNKAI OF KATA
SHIN GI TAI: KARATE TRAINING FOR BODY, MIND, AND SPIRIT
SIMPLE CHINESE MEDICINE
SIMPLE QIGONG EXERCISES FOR HEALTH, 3RD ED.
SIMPLIFIED TAI CHI CHUAN, 2ND ED.
SIMPLIFIED TAI CHI FOR BEGINNERS
SOLO TRAINING
SOLO TRAINING 2
SUDDEN DAWN: THE EPIC JOURNEY OF BODHIDHARMA
SUNRISE TAI CHI
SUNSET TAI CHI
SURVIVING ARMED ASSAULTS
TAE KWON DO: THE KOREAN MARTIAL ART
TAEKWONDO BLACK BELT POOMSAE
TAEKWONDO: A PATH TO EXCELLENCE
TAEKWONDO: ANCIENT WISDOM FOR THE MODERN WARRIOR
TAEKWONDO: DEFENSES AGAINST WEAPONS
TAEKWONDO: SPIRIT AND PRACTICE
TAO OF BIOENERGETICS
TAI CHI BALL QIGONG: FOR HEALTH AND MARTIAL ARTS
TAI CHI BALL WORKOUT FOR BEGINNERS
TAI CHI BOOK
TAI CHI CHIN NA: THE SEIZING ART OF TAI CHI CHUAN, 2ND ED.
TAI CHI CHUAN CLASSICAL YANG STYLE, 2ND ED.
TAI CHI CHUAN MARTIAL APPLICATIONS
TAI CHI CHUAN MARTIAL POWER, 3RD ED.
TAI CHI CONNECTIONS
TAI CHI DYNAMICS
TAI CHI QIGONG, 3RD ED.
TAI CHI SECRETS OF THE ANCIENT MASTERS
TAI CHI SECRETS OF THE WU & LI STYLES
TAI CHI SECRETS OF THE WU STYLE
TAI CHI SECRETS OF THE YANG STYLE
TAI CHI SWORD: CLASSICAL YANG STYLE, 2ND ED.
TAI CHI SWORD FOR BEGINNERS
TAI CHI WALKING
TAIJIQUAN THEORY OF DR. YANG, JWING-MING
TENGU: THE MOUNTAIN GOBLIN, A CONNOR BURKE MARTIAL ARTS THRILLER
TIMING IN THE FIGHTING ARTS
TRADITIONAL CHINESE HEALTH SECRETS
TRADITIONAL TAEKWONDO
TRAINING FOR SUDDEN VIOLENCE
WAY OF KATA
WAY OF KENDO AND KENJITSU
WAY OF SANCHIN KATA
WAY TO BLACK BELT
WESTERN HERBS FOR MARTIAL ARTISTS
WILD GOOSE QIGONG
WOMAN'S QIGONG GUIDE
XINGYIQUAN

DVDS FROM YMAA

ADVANCED PRACTICAL CHIN NA IN-DEPTH

ANALYSIS OF SHAOLIN CHIN NA

ATTACK THE ATTACK

BAGUAZHANG: EMEI BAGUAZHANG

CHEN STYLE TAIJIQUAN

CHIN NA IN-DEPTH COURSES 1—4

CHIN NA IN-DEPTH COURSES 5—8

CHIN NA IN-DEPTH COURSES 9—12

FACING VIOLENCE: 7 THINGS A MARTIAL ARTIST MUST KNOW

FIVE ANIMAL SPORTS

JOINT LOCKS

KNIFE DEFENSE: TRADITIONAL TECHNIQUES AGAINST A DAGGER

KUNG FU BODY CONDITIONING 1

KUNG FU BODY CONDITIONING 2

KUNG FU FOR KIDS

KUNG FU FOR TEENS

INFIGHTING

LOGIC OF VIOLENCE

MERIDIAN QIGONG

NEIGONG FOR MARTIAL ARTS

NORTHERN SHAOLIN SWORD : SAN CAI JIAN, KUN WU JIAN, QI MEN JIAN

QIGONG MASSAGE

QIGONG FOR HEALING

QIGONG FOR LONGEVITY

QIGONG FOR WOMEN

SABER FUNDAMENTAL TRAINING

SAI TRAINING AND SEQUENCES

SANCHIN KATA: TRADITIONAL TRAINING FOR KARATE POWER

SHAOLIN KUNG FU FUNDAMENTAL TRAINING: COURSES 1 & 2

SHAOLIN LONG FIST KUNG FU: BASIC SEQUENCES

SHAOLIN LONG FIST KUNG FU: INTERMEDIATE SEQUENCES

SHAOLIN LONG FIST KUNG FU: ADVANCED SEQUENCES 1

SHAOLIN LONG FIST KUNG FU: ADVANCED SEQUENCES 2

SHAOLIN SABER: BASIC SEQUENCES

SHAOLIN STAFF: BASIC SEQUENCES

SHAOLIN WHITE CRANE GONG FU BASIC TRAINING: COURSES 1 & 2

SHAOLIN WHITE CRANE GONG FU BASIC TRAINING: COURSES 3 & 4

SHUAI JIAO: KUNG FU WRESTLING

SIMPLE QIGONG EXERCISES FOR ARTHRITIS RELIEF

SIMPLE QIGONG EXERCISES FOR BACK PAIN RELIEF

SIMPLIFIED TAI CHI CHUAN: 24 & 48 POSTURES

SIMPLIFIED TAI CHI FOR BEGINNERS 48

SUNRISE TAI CHI

SUNSET TAI CHI

SWORD: FUNDAMENTAL TRAINING

TAEKWONDO KORYO POOMSAE

TAI CHI BALL QIGONG: COURSES 1 & 2

TAI CHI BALL QIGONG: COURSES 3 & 4

TAI CHI BALL WORKOUT FOR BEGINNERS

TAI CHI CHUAN CLASSICAL YANG STYLE

TAI CHI CONNECTIONS

TAI CHI ENERGY PATTERNS

TAI CHI FIGHTING SET

TAI CHI PUSHING HANDS: COURSES 1 & 2

TAI CHI PUSHING HANDS: COURSES 3 & 4

TAI CHI SWORD: CLASSICAL YANG STYLE

TAI CHI SWORD FOR BEGINNERS

TAI CHI SYMBOL: YIN YANG STICKING HANDS

TAIJI & SHAOLIN STAFF: FUNDAMENTAL TRAINING

TAIJI CHIN NA IN-DEPTH

TAIJI 37 POSTURES MARTIAL APPLICATIONS

TAIJI SABER CLASSICAL YANG STYLE

TAIJI WRESTLING

TRAINING FOR SUDDEN VIOLENCE

UNDERSTANDING QIGONG 1: WHAT IS QI? • HUMAN QI CIRCULATORY SYSTEM

UNDERSTANDING QIGONG 2: KEY POINTS • QIGONG BREATHING

UNDERSTANDING QIGONG 3: EMBRYONIC BREATHING

UNDERSTANDING QIGONG 4: FOUR SEASONS QIGONG

UNDERSTANDING QIGONG 5: SMALL CIRCULATION

UNDERSTANDING QIGONG 6: MARTIAL QIGONG BREATHING

WHITE CRANE HARD & SOFT QIGONG

WUDANG KUNG FU: FUNDAMENTAL TRAINING

WUDANG SWORD

WUDANG TAIJIQUAN

XINGYIQUAN

YANG TAI CHI FOR BEGINNERS

YMAA 25 YEAR ANNIVERSARY DVD

more products available from . . .

YMAA Publication Center, Inc. 楊氏東方文化出版中心

1-800-669-8892 • info@ymaa.com • www.ymaa.com